LIVING ✳ WELL
WITH EPILEPSY II

REPORT
OF THE 2003 NATIONAL CONFERENCE
ON PUBLIC HEALTH AND EPILEPSY

Priorities for a Public Health Agenda on Epilepsy

American Epilepsy Society

The Centers for Disease Control and Prevention

Chronic Disease Directors

Epilepsy Foundation

National Association of Epilepsy Centers

This publication was supported by Conference Support Grant Number R13/CCR321256-01 from the Centers for Disease Control and Prevention (CDC). Its contents are solely the responsibility of the Epilepsy Foundation and do not necessarily reflect the official views of the CDC, the Department of Health and Human Services, or the federal government.

For more information about this report or for additional copies, please contact:

Epilepsy Foundation
4351 Garden City Drive
Landover, MD 20785
(800) 332-1000
http://www.epilepsyfoundation.org

For more information about specific program activities, please contact:

Centers for Disease Control and Prevention
National Center for Chronic Disease Prevention and Health Promotion
Mail Stop K-40
4770 Buford Highway NE
Atlanta, GA 30341-3717
(770) 488-5131
ccdinfo@cdc.gov
www.cdc/gov/nccdphp

American Epilepsy Society
342 North Main Street
West Hartford, CT 06117-2507
(860) 586-7505
www.aesnet.org

National Association of Epilepsy Centers
5775 Wayzata Boulevard
Minneapolis, MN 55416
(612) 525-4526
www.naecepilepsy.org

Chronic Disease Directors
201 Greensboro Drive, Suite 300
McLean, VA 22102
(703) 610-9033
www.chronicdisease.org

FROM THE CO-CHAIR

On July 30 and 31, 2003, 200 health professionals, government officials, and consumers gathered to develop a comprehensive public health strategy for epilepsy. The *Living Well with Epilepsy II* conference, held in Baltimore, Maryland, addressed the many psychosocial and medical aspects of epilepsy that patients continue to struggle with each day.

Significant progress has been made since the first *Living Well with Epilepsy* conference in 1997; education for researchers and consumers has increased, as well as the issuance of specific guidelines for surgery from the American Academy of Neurology. Epilepsy has been addressed by the Agency for Healthcare Research and Quality, and its role in Medicaid contracting has been examined. Most significantly, advances in epilepsy research have allowed for earlier identification of refractory patients, thus allowing for increased treatment options.

There is however, a great deal of work ahead of us. Recommendations outlined in this report will help to shape the public health agenda in regards to epilepsy. The recommendations address the scope of this much needed work, including the need for early recognition, diagnosis, and treatment; improved epidemiology and surveillance; advances in self-management; and improved quality of life and impacts and outcomes of epilepsy. Their clear and focused implementation over the next five years will allow patients to begin to truly live well with epilepsy.

I thank our co-sponsors for their efforts on the *Living Well with Epilepsy II* conference: the Centers for Disease Control and Prevention, the American Epilepsy Society, Chronic Disease Directors, and National Association of Epilepsy Centers. I also express a special thank you to my co-chair, Patricia Osborne Shafer, whose leadership in creating this comprehensive report has been invaluable. For those of us on the planning committee, Patty has been the driving force and inspiration that has made all of this possible. Her energy and passion has set the example for all of us. She has been a gentle taskmaster, kindly encouraging everyone to their best efforts. Without her, this conference and this manuscript would never have been completed. This document represents her final official duties as the Chair of the Epilepsy Foundation Professional Advisory Board. To me, it will serve as a fitting work to her distinguished efforts for the past decade on behalf of the Epilepsy Foundation and all people with epilepsy.

Gregory L. Barkley, MD

TABLE OF CONTENTS

I. EXECUTIVE SUMMARY 4

II. INTRODUCTION 6
    Epilepsy: A Serious, Life-Altering Chronic Condition..................6
    The Public Health Approach...6
    Progress Since the First *Living Well with Epilepsy* Conference 7

III. *LIVING WELL WITH EPILEPSY II* CONFERENCE 8
    Co-Sponsors and Participants..8
    Conference Goals..8
    The Charge to Conference Workgroups......................................8

IV. REVIEW AND RECOMMENDATIONS 10
    Workgroup A: Early Recognition, Diagnosis and Treatment 10
        Charge and Workgroup Speakers 10
        Background..10
        Priority Recommendations...................................12
    Workgroup B: Epidemiology and Surveillance...........................13
        Charge and Workgroup Speakers 13
        Background..14
        Priority Recommendations...................................16
    Workgroup C: Self-Management..17
        Charge and Workgroup Speakers 17
        Background..17
        Priority Recommendations...................................21
    Workgroup D: Quality of Life – Impact and Outcome...................21
        Charge and Workgroup Speakers 21
        Background..22
        Priority Recommendations...................................24

V. SUMMARY 26

VI. REFERENCES 27

VII. APPENDICES 31
    Appendix A: Complete Listing of Recommendations
        for the *Living Well with Epilepsy II* Conference.....31
    Appendix B: Activities Resulting from 1997 *Living Well
        with Epilepsy* Conference 37
    Appendix C: Conference Planning Committee, Speakers,
        and Participants..38
    Appendix D: Conference Agendas and Speakers........................45
    Appendix E: Practice Parameters and Resources
        for Epilepsy Care..47

I. EXECUTIVE SUMMARY

The public health of our nation is increasingly burdened by chronic illnesses. Seizures and epilepsy (also known as recurring seizures) is one of these chronic disorders that affects 2.3 million Americans each year, and many more family members, friends, and caregivers regardless of age, sex, and ethnicity. With the changing demographics of the United States, the faces of epilepsy are changing – seizures can begin at any age, yet they occur most commonly in children and the elderly, with new-onset seizures in older Americans fast outpacing any other segment of our society. Seizures are a common neurological problem that, unfortunately, is under-recognized and not treated as significant by large segments of our society. It is commonly misunderstood because it is a collection of disorders that have different causes, consequences, and outcomes. For many people, epilepsy can be a self-limiting or easily controlled health problem, but for many more, epilepsy can be a life-long disorder requiring ongoing treatment and enormous resources to manage, cope with, and hopefully prevent, many disabling physical, social, cognitive, and emotional burdens.

Unfortunately, major deficiencies in our national approach to managing epilepsy are present, including the lack of an agreed upon protocol for aggressive control. Many people accept lack of seizure control as inevitable, and physicians too often subscribe to a similar philosophy. Consequently, people may never be referred to specialists or, when they are, many years of uncontrolled seizures may have already occurred. Although logic dictates that better, earlier care will result in better outcomes, research is needed to substantiate this hypothesis. Efforts to interrupt, prevent and change the development of epilepsy must be made with earlier, more aggressive, and systematic care. We must have systems and models of care that work better for people with epilepsy and allow people access to this care – people in rural America must have the same expectations and outcomes as those in urban America. Since epilepsy affects so many aspects of life, we must also assure that people obtain the necessary non-medical services needed to combat these problems.

Seizures and epilepsy, however, have only been recognized by the Centers for Disease Control and Prevention as a public health concern for the past 10 years, and, although epilepsy is clearly a chronic disease with both medical and social components, it has not been a public health priority. This was partly because public health has traditionally focused on tracking sources of infectious disease and related health hazards with a view to controlling and preventing their effects and promoting a more healthy society. However, as medical care extends the lives of the chronically ill, their issues are increasingly affecting the social fabric and the character of public health. The need to track the incidence, prevalence, mortality, health status, quality of life, and social outcomes of chronic disease is now more pressing, requiring the public health community to pay greater attention to these issues, using many of the same strategies with which they formerly tracked infection and its management.

In 1997, the Centers for Disease Control and Prevention, together with key thought leaders and stakeholders, began crafting a public health agenda to target key challenges facing people with epilepsy. Despite substantial efforts, the epilepsy and public health communities have recognized a continuing lack of awareness regarding the seriousness of epilepsy and available treatment options among people with epilepsy, health care professionals, and the general public. Delays and discrepancies in how epilepsy and its consequences are manifested, diagnosed and treated persist, and are complicated by the social and cultural complexities of our society. These issues led to the need to re-examine critical issues associated with epilepsy and how the public health community can respond most effectively to them.

Living Well with Epilepsy II, a national conference on public health and epilepsy, was held in July 2003, and brought invited experts from the medical, public health, academic, advocacy, voluntary health, and corporate communities together with people with epilepsy and their families. The goal of the conference was clear – review progress since the first *Living Well with Epilepsy* conference, recommend needs and priorities for a public health agenda on epilepsy for the next five years, and identify other challenges that must be addressed by the epilepsy community and those who support it. Participants were assigned to explore one of four areas – Early Recognition, Diagnosis, and Treatment; Epidemiology and Surveillance; Self-Management; and Quality of Life – Impact and Outcomes – and asked to address the following tasks:

- **To review recent progress** in the understanding of seizures and epilepsy.

- **To identify critical gaps** in the scientific basis for effective recognition, treatment, and prevention of epilepsy and its co-morbidities, including effects on cognition and mood.

- **To recommend policies and strategies** for removing barriers to optimal health and functioning for persons with seizures and epilepsy, including attitudinal barriers within society.

Key themes from the
Living Well with Epilepsy II conference

Several recommendations emerged from this conference that chart a course for the public health community. The body of this report offers recommendations identified as priority areas by workgroup participants; however, many more needs and recommendations were identified and can be found in Appendix A. Although this conference focused on public health, the conference planning committee hopes that other federal and state agencies and everyone who supports and cares for people with seizures and epilepsy will look at these needs and see where their efforts can make a difference. The priority conference recommendations highlight the following themes:

- There is a critical need for improved access to epilepsy specialists and comprehensive systems of epilepsy care and to improve the early detection and treatment of seizures.

- Establishing criteria for quality care in epilepsy and for the co-morbidities that may accompany it is urgently needed.

- Substantial gaps exist in our current understanding, including diagnosis and treatment of epilepsy's consequences, especially in the areas of mental health and cognition.

- Systems and models of care must foster empowerment and independence for people with epilepsy and support their efforts towards improved seizure control and a positive quality of life.

- Surveillance systems must address critical issues for people with epilepsy, including the burden of disease, mortality risks, and a firmer picture of its incidence and prevalence, particularly in special populations.

- Stigma remains a major barrier to effective awareness, care, and quality of life and requires new research and communication approaches to combat it.

- Public education is critical to improving seizure recognition and first aid, the hallmarks of early detection and treatment of people with seizures.

America has the capacity to prevent or mitigate many of the untoward consequences of epilepsy, but change, ambitious efforts, and persistence are needed to accomplish this. The conference sponsors believe that the time has come for this to occur. As Tony Coelho, chair-elect of the Epilepsy Foundation board of directors declared, "What have we learned? They won't do something for us unless we ask, not unless we push to help ourselves... When we walk out this door, we should not only agree on our ideas, but we should do something about it. Epilepsy *is* an urgent topic. I challenge you...to implement what we have discussed. Everything that was said is doable. It takes money. It takes work. It takes coordination. It takes passion. *We can and must do it!*"

I. INTRODUCTION

A. Epilepsy: A Serious, Life-Altering, Chronic Condition

Epilepsy is a common neurological disorder marked by involuntary, recurrent seizures that arise from excessive discharges of neurons in the brain. Seizures vary in type, severity and intensity, and can be manifested by changes in consciousness, movement, sensation, or behavior. Based on 1995 data, seizures and epilepsy are estimated to affect approximately 2.3 million people with 181,000 new cases per year in the United States (1). By age 85, approximately 10% of the population will have experienced at least one unprovoked or acute symptomatic seizure and 4% will have developed epilepsy (2).

Epilepsy — that is, the occurrence of more than one unprovoked seizure — affects both men and women, yet gender-specific patterns have been noted. Females develop seizures at greater rates in the first five years of life, but males predominate after this age, with the greatest differences noted in the older age groups (2). While seizures may begin at any age, children and the elderly are most susceptible. Epilepsy syndromes of childhood include some of the most devastating forms of the condition, changing young lives forever. And although epilepsy is a physical disorder of brain function, it carries with it a substantial social burden that expresses itself in high rates of unemployment, personal isolation, and the stigma of "spoiled identity" (3).

Available treatment options include antiepileptic drugs, surgery, vagus nerve stimulation, and the ketogenic diet, but large gaps in access to care are apparent, especially access to secondary and tertiary level care. It is not unusual for several years to pass before an individual receives a precise diagnosis and treatment. It has been estimated that more than 40% of the population with epilepsy continue to have seizures, while many others pay a heavy price in side effects from treatment (1).

Epilepsy can be a self-limiting disease or one that is readily treatable if diagnosed properly; however, for too many people it is a lifetime condition, resulting in substantial morbidity and increased mortality. Co-morbidities in the form of cognitive difficulties and depressed mood add to its burden. The annual cost to society is estimated at $12.5 billion (in 1995 dollars), of which 85% are indirect costs (3). In 2000, Begley and colleagues reported that "epilepsy is unique among chronic conditions in terms of the relatively high percentage of indirect morbidity-related costs, 70% for persons with intractable epilepsy… compared with an average of 11% for all persons with chronic disease (1)." Despite its impact on the individual and society, epilepsy remains a hidden disorder, difficult to quantify and, until recently, largely absent from the nation's public health agenda.

B. The Public Health Approach

For many years, epilepsy, though clearly a chronic disease with both medical and social components, was not a public health priority. This was partly because public health has traditionally focused on tracking sources of infectious disease and related health hazards with a view to controlling and preventing their effects and promoting a more healthy society. However, as medical care extends the lives of the chronically ill, their issues are increasingly affecting the social fabric and the character of public health. The need to track the incidence, prevalence, health status, quality of life, and social outcomes of chronic disease is now more pressing, requiring the public health community to pay ever greater attention to these issues, using many of the same strategies with which they formerly tracked infection and its management.

During the past decade, the public health community, through the work of the Centers for Disease Control and Prevention (CDC), has been paying increasing attention to epilepsy: its epidemiology, diagnosis, and treatment, and the importance of improved public awareness. The core functions of public health – assessment, policy development, and assurance – are being used to improve knowledge and understanding of epilepsy's impact on society and the individual and to develop a series of strategic, evidence-based responses to the condition.

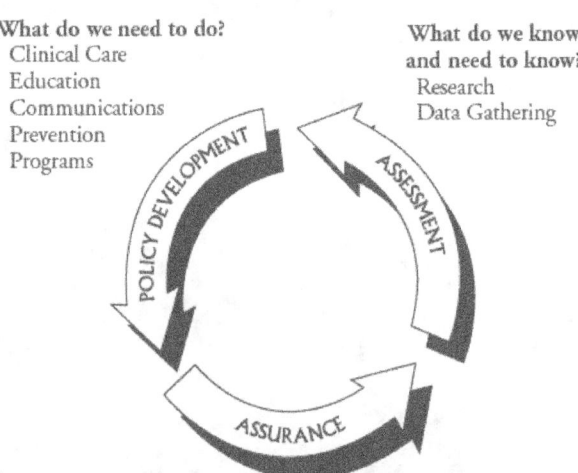

What do we need to do?
Clinical Care
Education
Communications
Prevention
Programs

What do we know and need to know?
Research
Data Gathering

Making sure it's done well
Evaluation
Measuring Outcomes

The *assessment* function of public health is applied to determine what data are needed to identify and address core problems associated with epilepsy and seizures, using epidemiological and surveillance systems to monitor the extent to which epilepsy affects Americans and the health outcomes experienced by those who have it. *Policy development* is a key public health function that uses assessment information to identify and promote effective programs, services, and health care delivery systems needed for the care of people with epilepsy, and to identify corrective policies and action plans that eliminate barriers to successful care. The *assurance* function of public health is similarly vital to make certain that patients with epilepsy and their families are getting the programs and services they need to effectively manage the challenges of living with an unpredictable, episodic neurological disorder such as epilepsy.

In 1994, the National Center for Chronic Disease Prevention and Health Promotion for the first time convened a group of experts representing the epilepsy treatment and advocacy communities to help the agency shape a public health agenda for epilepsy. Three years later, it sponsored the first major public health conference on epilepsy, with the theme of *Living Well with Epilepsy*. That meeting was organized around the core functions of public health, and it produced a series of recommendations to use as a blueprint for the public health response to epilepsy in the years ahead.

C. Progress Since the First *Living Well with Epilepsy* Conference

The first *Living Well with Epilepsy* conference defined the goal of epilepsy treatment as "No Seizures, No Side Effects." Its key message to the health care community was summarized as: "take seizures seriously; do it early and do it right the first time; be systematic, efficient and effective; and empower the patient." It also urged greater attention to the role of stigma as a major component of epilepsy's social burden, as well as a key barrier to accessing care and developing effective self-management behaviors. As a result of these and the many other recommendations that came out of the conference, the CDC has collaborated with government agencies, academic centers, and national organizations to initiate and strengthen many program activities in the field of epilepsy. These activities include:

- Collaboration with the Agency for Healthcare Research and Quality (AHRQ) to assess the evidence linking elements of care to clinical outcomes in special populations of patients with epilepsy;

- Collaboration with the George Washington University Center for Health Services Research and

Policy on development of health service purchasing specifications for services related to epilepsy;

- Collaboration with the Epilepsy Foundation to enhance awareness and understanding of epilepsy through targeted education and awareness campaigns and increased support of research;

- Development of a bibliography/database of work related to epilepsy self-management;

- Support of initiatives at two CDC Prevention Research Centers (academic research centers housed within schools of public health and medicine) to implement and evaluate self-management interventions in epilepsy;

- Support of population-based epidemiological studies of epilepsy prevalence, incidence, and healthcare needs in selected communities;

- Assessment of the utility of existing health care data sets for studying trends in access to care, levels of care, and other demographic variables related to epilepsy;

- Continuing development of a tool to assess public perceptions of epilepsy;

- Support of epidemiological studies of preventable causes of epilepsy, including traumatic brain injury and infections such as cysticercosis, a common, preventable cause of epilepsy;

- Evaluation of the incidence, prevalence and patterns of care for epilepsy in a managed care setting.

(See Appendix B for a complete listing of resources and activities developed as a result of the first *Living Well with Epilepsy* conference.)

Despite these substantial efforts, the epilepsy and public health communities have recognized a continuing lack of awareness regarding the seriousness of epilepsy and available treatment options among people with epilepsy, health care professionals, and the general public. Delays and discrepancies in how epilepsy and its consequences are manifested, diagnosed, and treated persist, and are complicated by the social and cultural complexities of our society. These issues led to the need to re-examine critical issues associated with epilepsy and how the public health community can respond most effectively to them.

III. *LIVING WELL WITH EPILEPSY II* CONFERENCE

A. Co-Sponsors and Participants

Living Well with Epilepsy II, the second national conference on public health and epilepsy, was held July 30-31, 2003, in Baltimore, Maryland. Co-sponsored by CDC, the American Epilepsy Society (AES), the Chronic Disease Directors (CDD), the National Association of Epilepsy Centers (NAEC), and the Epilepsy Foundation, the conference brought together:

- specialists in the public health disciplines of prevention, epidemiology, health education, and health promotion

- clinicians who treat persons with epilepsy and scientists engaged in research

- other health care professionals

- advocates for persons with epilepsy and their families

- representatives of health care delivery systems and organizations

- people with epilepsy and their families

(Conference planning committee, participants and contributors are identified in Appendix C.)

B. Conference Goals

Conference participants shared common constituencies, research interests, and a strong commitment to improving the lives of people with epilepsy. The co-sponsors brought this community of interest together to review progress since the first *Living Well with Epilepsy* conference, recommend needs and priorities for a public health agenda on epilepsy for the next five years, and identify other challenges that must be addressed by the epilepsy community and those who support it.

Participants addressed the following tasks:

- **To review recent progress** in the understanding of seizures and epilepsy.

- **To identify critical gaps** in the scientific basis for effective recognition, treatment, and prevention of epilepsy and its co-morbidities, including effects on cognition and mood.

- **To recommend policies and strategies** for removing barriers to optimal health and functioning for persons with seizures and epilepsy, including attitudinal barriers within society.

C. The Charge to Conference Workgroups

The conference planning committee organized the meeting into four workgroups, closely paralleling the core functions of public health.

- **Group A: Early Recognition, Diagnosis and Treatment** – designed to promote policy development through identification of clinical issues and priority questions for clinical research.

- **Group B: Epidemiology and Surveillance** – to assess epilepsy's impact through examination of current data systems , appropriate surveillance and data collection, and the identification of measurement gaps.

- **Group C: Self-Management** – to assure that people with epilepsy have the information and support they need to manage the condition and its treatment effectively.

- **Group D: Quality of Life – Impact and Outcomes** – to identify issues which negatively affect quality of life in those with epilepsy and assure improvements through development of effective policies, programs, communication strategies, and interventions.

In addition, each workgroup was asked to consider epilepsy in a broader context, viewing seizures as a spectrum of disorders with diverse causes, consequences, and prognoses that vary with age, gender, and ethnicity, and to discuss how these factors may affect the organization of care for people with epilepsy.

The conference began with a plenary session in which members of the epilepsy and public health communities reviewed the public health approach to epilepsy since the first conference, and outlined potential opportunities for the future. The participants then met in their assigned workgroups to examine these topics in relation to the core functions of public health, and to deliberate on key issues previously identified by the planning committee for each group. Workgroup sessions were organized around brief presentations that addressed critical themes or problems. Reactors (experts chosen for their insight and expertise from other disciplines or constituencies) responded to the expert presentations, highlighting areas for participants to consider in their deliberations or offering examples of relevant incidents, experiences, or programs. (A list of workgroup agendas, presenters, and respondents appear in Appendix D.)

Formal recommendations for action on the part of the CDC, its partners in public health, and the broader epilepsy community were arrived at by vote of each of the four workgroups. In each case, participants first deliberated in small breakout groups organized around key issues for discussion, as previously outlined in the expert presentations. Members of these small groups were assigned to assure a balance of interest between health professionals, representatives of the public health community, consumers, and advocates. Each small group prioritized its recommendations by vote and reported these to the workgroup, which noted areas of consensus or priority as determined by the small groups. Additionally, the co-chairs of each group synthesized its recommendations, and identified common themes. Co-chairs presented their groups' priority recommendations at the conclusion of the meeting, and these form the body of this report. Subsequently, the recommendations were cross-referenced with written and audio transcripts of the proceedings. Several workgroups identified similar needs and made similar recommendations, leading to consolidation where appropriate. To avoid repetition, recommendations in this report made by more than one workgroup are identified in parenthesis, by workgroup letter. In the interests of reflecting the whole range of needed actions identified by the small groups during discussions, the latter are reported in Appendix A.

IV. REVIEW AND RECOMMENDATIONS

Workgroup A
Early Recognition, Diagnosis, and Treatment

A. Charge

Workgroup A was charged to examine the following issues:

- Is there an agreed upon standard of optimal care for the treatment of epilepsy along the spectrum of the disorder (e.g. new-onset seizures, well-controlled epilepsy, or seizures that persist or are intractable despite treatment) and do these represent the consensus of experts in the field of epilepsy?

- How do the expectations of patients, primary care physicians, general neurologists, and insurers differ from epilepsy experts with respect to the provision of optimal therapy for epilepsy?

- What tools are needed by patients, families, and caregivers to take ownership of their epilepsy care and enable them to adequately evaluate the care and determine if changes in treatment are warranted?

- How can systems of care address quality of care issues in the diagnosis and treatment of seizures and epilepsy, including critical non-physician services?

- How can disparities in the quality of care between resource-rich and resource-poor systems be alleviated, providing patients greater access to quality care?

B. Workgroup Speakers

Participants in this workgroup were asked to discuss early recognition, diagnosis, and treatment of seizures and epilepsy, framed by the preceding questions, and to develop appropriate strategies. Critical issues and challenges facing participants, presented by the following experts, were used in addition to related sources for the following background information.

Presenters
- Recognition and diagnosis: Gregory L. Holmes, MD, Dartmouth Hitchcock Medical Center, and Susan Axelrod, Citizens United for Research in Epilepsy
- Access to care and treatment: Jacqueline A. French, MD, University of Pennsylvania, and Susan Eik Filstead, The Susan Eik Filstead Stroke and Epilepsy Foundation

Reactors
- Santi K.M. Bhaghat, MD, Potomac, Maryland
- John Booss, MD, Veterans Administration Connecticut Healthcare Systems
- Jeffrey Levi, PhD, George Washington University Medical Center
- Suzanne M. Smith, MD, Centers for Disease Control and Prevention

C. Background

Improving detection and diagnosis

Technological and genetic advances are improving the ability of health care professionals to diagnose seizures and epilepsy, while researchers are evaluating new ways to predict or stop seizures and to identify those who are likely to respond to medical therapy. However, for too many people epilepsy remains overlooked or misdiagnosed. Unfortunately, delayed diagnosis results in patients receiving inappropriate or ineffective care for years, and places them at risk for developing refractory seizures, secondary disabilities, and related problems (4).

A diagnosis of epilepsy is based on the clinical history and descriptions of events. However, diagnostic tests are needed to determine the presence and location of epileptiform activity, possible causes, and the impact of seizures on brain function, all of which may influence treatment and prognosis (5). While evidence is sparse on the strengths of different diagnostic tests, a complete history and physical examination with neuropsychological assessment and routine electroencephalograms (EEG), are indicated to diagnose epilepsy. Imaging studies and video EEG may be needed to determine causes of seizures and confirm difficult diagnostic situations (6). More detailed testing is necessary when a person's seizures are not responding to treatment as expected, or other treatment alternatives must be considered. Further research is essential to evaluate the benefits and outcomes of diagnostic testing at different stages of epilepsy (e.g. new-onset and intractable).

Improving care to people with seizures requires acknowledging the need for enhanced seizure recognition, access to medical expertise and resources, and access to treatments. An expansion of clinical research is also critical to understanding the needs and outcomes in distinct population groups and at different points along epilepsy's continuum of severity. However, enhancing awareness of seizures and epilepsy is the first step to progress in any of these areas. Surveys have indicated a lack of awareness of seizures and basic first aid among adolescents and adults without epilepsy (7, 8) as well as lack of knowledge among selected groups of health care professionals regarding care of women with epilepsy (9, 10). This lack of awareness contributes to delays in recognition and treatment. While educational efforts have been undertaken in selected communities served by Epilepsy Foundation affiliates or epilepsy specialists, these efforts have not been systematically disseminated, implemented, or evaluated. Expanding educational endeavors must focus on improving recognition, diagnosis, and care of seizures, and be particularly targeted to reaching those who are likely to be points of first contact for people with new-onset seizures.

Treating epilepsy as a serious health problem

Discrepancies exist as to the seriousness of epilepsy, in part because epilepsy is not a single disorder, but a group of disorders with different etiologies, manifestations, and prognoses. In an incident-based cost of illness study, Begley and colleagues (1) found that 25% of those with new-onset seizures were likely to develop persistent seizures that do not respond to standard medical therapy. Recent work by Kwan and Brodie (11, 4) categorized people according to those who are treatment-responsive and those who are treatment-resistant and suggested that the first antiepileptic drug (AED) used will control seizures in 47% of people with newly diagnosed epilepsy and an additional 13% will become seizure free with the second AED tried. These data reinforce the finding that if seizures are treated early and appropriately, many people will do well, but a significant number will progress to a life of chronic, persistent seizures with far-reaching outcomes.

Predictors of persistent seizures are still not completely understood; however, certain epilepsy syndromes or seizure types are more likely to become intractable and lead to adverse consequences and disability. For example, children with infantile spasms are more likely to develop Lennox-Gastaut syndrome (12), a progressive disorder that includes refractory seizures, cognitive decline, and functional and behavioral deterioration. Those with a symptomatic cause of seizures, such as head trauma, tumor, or infection, also are more likely to experience recurrent seizures (13). Additionally, recent research suggests that a genetic alteration may play a role in determining whether patients respond to AEDs (14).

The ability to better identify responders, as well as determine more precise timing and implementation of treatment, may help prevent the development of refractory epilepsy (15). For example, people identified as having benign epilepsy syndromes or seizure types may not need aggressive, long-term treatment. For others, access to an experienced neurologist or epileptologist may be critical to ensure that they are properly diagnosed and medications chosen appropriately, especially when they are unresponsive to their first or second AED, when women are planning a pregnancy, or when discontinuation of AEDs is under consideration. People who do not respond to initial medical therapy should have access to all other therapies, such as rational AED polytherapy, epilepsy surgery, vagus nerve stimulation, or the ketogenic diet (16). The effectiveness, risks and costs of different therapies need further study, particularly in relation to different population groups and long-term consequences, since most people remain on the first one or two AEDs tried.

Choosing medications for epilepsy can be complicated by factors such as age, seizure type and/or syndrome, presence of co-morbid conditions, allergies, dosing interval, titration rate, formulations, short and long term adverse effects, teratogenicity, and cost (17). A recently published practice parameter regarding the efficacy and tolerability of AEDs in new-onset epilepsy suggests that both standard AEDs and many of the newer AEDs can be used, with the choice of drug dependent on patient characteristics (18). The evidence for use of the newer AEDs in refractory epilepsy is less clear, but the parameter offers guidelines for use of the AEDs by tailoring treatment to seizure, safety, and patient characteristics (19). Additionally, a randomized controlled trial of epilepsy surgery patients suggests that temporal lobe resections in those who are appropriate candidates for surgery offer greater freedom from disabling seizures and greater improvement in quality of life than chronic medical therapy alone (20). Yet it is critical that we have better data regarding the long-term consequences and impact on quality of life in distinct groups and use this data to identify predictors of success.

Making informed decisions regarding treatment alternatives requires that health care providers and people with epilepsy understand and appreciate the risks and seriousness of their disorder. Seizures are often, and sometimes mistakenly, considered benign symptoms, yet for too many people seizures end in death. The need for enhanced epidemiological studies to better understand the causes of death in epilepsy is critical (see Workgroup B). At the same time however, people must learn how to assess their risks and pursue appropriate strategies that may prevent epilepsy-related deaths. Unfortunately, mortality in epilepsy is not easily talked about or incorporated into educational programs. Support systems for grieving families are sparse. These gaps must be rectified so that health care professionals and people with epilepsy and their families obtain much needed education and help, and that potentially devastating consequences of epilepsy are acknowledged and addressed appropriately.

Unfortunately, cost has become a major factor in access to treatment. The cost varies dramatically when the newer AEDs are compared to the "old" and medical treatment is compared to surgical approaches (21). Evidence suggests that most of the newer drugs are better tolerated, making them easier and safer to use in many situations (20). However, additional research is clearly needed to explore the economic consequences of seizures and economic benefits of timely, effective treatment and prevention of secondary disability.

In addition to the need for further research, patients and health care professionals must have access to current guidelines and best practices for treatment and provision of services to improve the quality of care rendered. Practice parameters have been published on the diagnosis of seizures in selected populations, care of women with epilepsy, surgical treatment, and use of AEDs, as well as optional purchasing specifications for epilepsy services (see Appendix E) (22, 23). However, for real practice changes to occur, enhanced efforts must be devoted to disseminating these documents to the medical community and consumers. Experts and consumers can then devote effort to defining optimal care in epilepsy, and establishing 'road maps' and educational materials that will facilitate access to quality care for consumers. This information can guide providers and insurers in appropriate referral patterns and coverage of necessary services.

Healthcare resources

People newly diagnosed with seizures may receive treatment from a pediatrician, primary care physician, or emergency room physician who, at times, may consult with a neurologist or epileptologist. However, an epilepsy specialist is rarely the first medical professional to initiate treatment. When diagnosis or treatment is difficult, evaluation by a neurologist specializing in epilepsy or by an epilepsy center is often necessary to ensure that the diagnosis is correct and that appropriate treatment is initiated as early as possible after diagnosis (23).

There remain major deficiencies in our national approach to managing epilepsy, including the lack of an agreed upon protocol for aggressive control. Many patients accept lack of seizure control as inevitable, and physicians too often subscribe to a similar philosophy. Consequently, patients may never be referred to specialists or, when they are, many years of uncontrolled seizures may have already occurred. Berg and colleagues (24) found that of 333 patients with partial epilepsy followed prospectively, the average time from seizure onset to failure of a second drug was nine years, with younger age of onset being the most significant predictor. This highlights a fact that many clinicians have known for too long – people are waiting too long to get the care they need. While it may take years to develop treatment resistant epilepsy, delays in referral to specialists or lack of access to care may exacerbate this dilemma. After so many years of living with chronic seizures, successful adjustment to life with a job, family, and social responsibilities may be impossible.

Unfortunately, resources for epilepsy care are limited. Unpublished data from the National Association of Epilepsy Centers suggests that there are approximately 600 neurologists in the United States who specialize in epilepsy. There is also a worsening shortage of pediatric neurologists, which limits the availability of specialized medical expertise. While common diagnostic tests (e.g. EEGs and MRIs) are available in major hospitals, more advanced testing such as positron emission tomography (PET), single photon emission computed tomography (SPECT), and magnetoencephalography (MEG) tend to be available only at specialized academic centers. Access to approved therapies, including many AEDs, the vagus nerve stimulator, and epilepsy surgery are subject to limitations imposed by availability, willingness of the health professional to refer for specialized treatment, or to financial limitations due to insufficient insurance coverage.

Better care, better outcomes

Although logic dictates that better, earlier care will result in better outcomes, research is needed to substantiate this hypothesis. Can the development of epilepsy be interrupted, prevented, and changed if care is obtained earlier, more aggressively, and systematically? A randomized trial of 'customary care' versus early referral to a specialist is critical to explore the benefits, costs, and feasibility of different models of care. Levels of providing care and models of shared or collaborative care have become increasing popular in other countries, but their effectiveness in treating epilepsy has not been systematically examined in the United States. In particular, research is needed to determine whether recognizing seizures early and providing appropriate diagnostic testing and treatment improves the outcomes of care and prevents secondary morbidity and mortality.

D. Priority Recommendations: Early Recognition, Diagnosis and Treatment

Participants in this workgroup formulated their recommendations on the need for research, policies, and practices/programs to improve seizure recognition, diagnosis, and treatment. The following includes the priority recommendations consolidated under major themes explored in this group. Additional recommendations can be found in Appendix A:

1. **Support research to evaluate existing best practices and standards of care for persons with epilepsy.**
   a. Support and encourage health services and outcomes research to evaluate the impact of various levels and types of epilepsy care, including critical non-physician services and education.
   b. Support a randomized trial of 'customary care' versus early referral to specialized care.
   c. Support clinical research to evaluate the long-term benefits, risks, and costs of all treatment alternatives for seizures and epilepsy, including the risks and benefits of treatments on learning, cognition, and health-related quality of life (HRQOL).

2. **Improve understanding of seizures and epilepsy and best practices for epilepsy management, including referral to tertiary level of care, particularly for primary care providers.**
   a. Develop consensus on definitions and indicators of quality care for epilepsy.
   b. Enhance communication and dissemination of standards of care and best practices among health care professionals, the public health community, health plans/insurers, people with epilepsy, and families.
   c. Undertake a "living with epilepsy" campaign to empower people with epilepsy and professionals to work aggressively towards the goals of 'no seizures and no side effects.' Incorporate information on patient and family expectations and rights, guidelines and indicators of quality care, how to access care, and community resources for epilepsy education and support.

3. **Improve early recognition and timely diagnosis of seizures and epilepsy, including rare forms of seizures.**
   a. Develop and implement public awareness and education campaigns on seizure recognition and diagnosis targeted to first responders, school personnel, and health care professionals.
   b. Enhance dissemination of educational materials to emergency rooms, diagnostic laboratories, mental health clinics, and primary health care sites.
   c. Enhance efforts to survey the general public's awareness, attitudes, and knowledge of epilepsy, including perceived barriers to seizure recognition and diagnosis.

4. **Improve access to optimal care for persons with epilepsy.**
   a. Conduct demonstration projects to improve access to care in both urban and rural areas and among diverse population groups.
   b. Replicate successful community programs that promote early recognition, timely diagnosis, and access to appropriate care, particularly to underserved geographical areas and groups.
   c. Improve the availability of specialized comprehensive care nationwide and encourage practices and systems that support comprehensive epilepsy care.

5. **Improve recognition and use of appropriate seizure first aid.**
   a. Develop consensus criteria on the warning signs of seizures and epilepsy.
   b. Develop and implement educational programs for the general public on the warning signs of seizures

to enhance early recognition.
   c. Support the development and dissemination of school-based epilepsy curricula to enhance seizure recognition and first aid.
   d. Promote universal teaching of appropriate seizure first aid as a component of standard first aid curriculums for schools and the general public.

6. **Enhance understanding of mortality in epilepsy among all audiences.**
   a. Develop educational materials and programs on death in epilepsy and preventable causes for professional and lay audiences.
   b. Incorporate the relationship of mortality to seizure severity and control in educational materials.
   c. Evaluate best practices to reduce mortality, particularly the impact of early intervention.
   d. Create support systems and resources for families and caregivers to assist in coping with epilepsy-related death.

Workgroup B
Epidemiology and Surveillance

A. Charge

Workgroup B was charged to examine the following issues:

- Systems and methods needed for improved surveillance of epilepsy in the United States, with specific attention to existing or new data sources; working case definitions; state capacity; and other approaches such as use of managed care organization data, registries, and geographic information systems.

- Preferred focus of epilepsy surveillance systems, with specific consideration of incidence, prevalence, patterns of care, subpopulations (e.g. age, gender, race/ethnicity) at increased risk, and secular trends.

- Priority of special epidemiological studies of epilepsy, with specific consideration of subpopulations at increased risk, access to primary and specialty care, epilepsy etiology, type and severity, quality of life issues, disability and co-morbidity, and cost.

- Appropriate division of responsibilities for addressing epilepsy surveillance and epidemiological research priorities among CDC, National Institutes of Health (NIH), other federal agencies and state health departments.

B. Workgroup Speakers

Key areas to be addressed during the workgroup were presented by the following experts, followed by remarks from the reactor panel. The following background information is drawn from these presentations and related sources.

Presenters
- Overview of epidemiology and surveillance: W. Allen Hauser, MD, Columbia University
- Epilepsy in children: Edwin Trevathan, MD, MPH, Washington University School of Medicine
- Epilepsy in the elderly: R. Eugene Ramsay, MD, University of Miami School of Medicine
- Epilepsy in minority populations: Dale C. Hesdorffer, PhD, G.H. Sergievsky Center
- Socioeconomic status: Charles E. Begley, PhD, University of Texas School of Public Health
- Mortality in epilepsy: Michael R. Sperling, MD, Thomas Jefferson University Hospital

Reactors
- Linda D. Lanier, The Sarcoidosis Awareness Network
- Anbesaw W. Selassie, DrPH, Medical University of South Carolina
- David Thurman, MD, MPH, Centers for Disease Control and Prevention
- Marshalynn Yeargin-Allsopp, MD, Centers for Disease Control and Prevention

C. Background

Epidemiology is the study of patterns of disease occurrence in human populations and the factors that influence these patterns. Such studies are crucial to understand the determinants of illness (e.g. patient characteristics, patterns of occurrence, potential causes), the determinants of outcome (e.g. mortality, remission, co-morbid conditions), and potential costs. The ultimate goal of epidemiology/surveillance research is prevention. Population studies frequently report the incidence of epilepsy, which is the number of new cases during a defined period of time, within a limited geographical area and defined population. Prevalence describes the number of active cases at a point in time. Prevalence data serves to define society's burden of illness, which can lead to the allocation of appropriate funding and health care resources. The estimated prevalence of epilepsy is complicated by what we do not know, such as the influence of mortality and remission. For example, current prevalence in children has been estimated at 7.7/1000 (25) and in the general population at around 10/1000 (1). These and similar estimates rely on projection of data gathered in scattered areas of the country. Currently three com-

munity level surveys suggest a higher prevalence of 1.7 – 2.6% (26, 27). The true prevalence of epilepsy in the United States remains unknown, partly because the terms "seizures, seizure disorder/epilepsy" are not currently included in public health data collection systems. This should be remedied and studies to establish true incidence and prevalence rates should be undertaken without delay.

For epilepsy, it is equally important to understand determinants of the illness and its outcomes, and ultimately to succeed in its prevention. Priorities include the development of surveillance systems to assess the incidence of new cases, patterns of care and the presence of co-morbid conditions, seizure and epilepsy-associated mortality, and current and planned data sources. Surveillance is particularly important in special populations. Little is known about the incidence, prevalence and impact of epilepsy among those living in rural areas, people of low socioeconomic status, Spanish-speaking populations, African Americans, Asians, Native Americans, those with developmental disabilities or psychiatric disorders, and other distinct population groups. Most studies compare blacks to whites, and only one has data on Hispanics. Multipoint identification in an epilepsy surveillance system could include sites of first or frequent contact for people with seizures, such as physicians' offices and clinics, emergency rooms, laboratory facilities providing EEG and MRI services, and nursing homes, as well as state and local government health and social service agencies.

The ability to track cases from time of first identification is of primary importance and will bolster currently limited information on epilepsy prognosis, mortality, presence and prevalence of other medical conditions, cost, and support. Epidemiological studies that are representative of the population of people with epilepsy, e.g. studies of incidence cohorts identified through surveillance programs, can help accomplish these goals, thus providing opportunities for prevention. Such studies must also include data on adverse events from AEDs or other treatments, as well as interactions between AEDs and other drugs or health conditions, and should correspond to the entire course of treatment.

Patterns of health care
Health care use varies with the stage of the disorder and prognosis. For example, Begley and colleagues (1) found that health care use in the first year after a diagnosis of epilepsy is 3-4 times greater than in subsequent years. Using 1995 estimates, hospitalizations account for 50-60% of epilepsy health care costs, with AEDs comprising only 20-30%. For people who achieve seizure control early, costs are greatest in the first three years. However, for those whose seizures persist, AED use actually increases and the decrease in outpatient visits is much less dramatic in the years that follow. Overall, people with active seizures use about 2-3 times more health care than those whose seizures are controlled, and the costs to them and to society increase

with each increment in seizure frequency. More important-
ly, the outcomes for those with active seizures differ from
those of people whose seizures are easily controlled. Total
costs are five times higher for those with active seizures,
with indirect costs (the negative impact of seizures on pro-
ductivity at work and at home) being the most significant
contributor to total costs. Understanding current patterns
of health care use and costs highlight the needs of different
groups with epilepsy, and, when looked at together with
outcomes, may suggest ways of improving systems of care
while managing resources and costs appropriately.

Assessment of patterns of care from time of first seizure
should include identification of providers, direct and indirect cost estimates, effects of delays in diagnosis and referral
to tertiary care, accuracy of diagnosis, and patterns of non-
medical care. In addition, data are needed on the prevalence of symptoms that resemble epileptic seizures, but are
actually manifestations of various psychiatric syndromes.
Known as psychogenic non-epileptic seizures, these are
often confused with or misidentified as epileptic seizures
and may confound survey data on epilepsy. It has been
suggested that non-epileptic seizures are present in 10 to 45
percent of patients with refractory epilepsy (28) with psychiatric issues (depression, anxiety, and obsession) involved
in many cases (29).

Epilepsy in children

Based on the 1995 population, there were an estimated
315,000 children with epilepsy under the age of 14 in the
United States, of whom 88,845 had severe and intractable
epilepsy (1). In one recent study, 220 children with epilepsy were followed for more than 20 years (30). The results
were sobering; 44 (20%) died, of whom 39 (89%) had persistent seizures. Ninety-three (53%) required medications
throughout the study and 76 (36%) were "refractory" or
non-responsive to standard medical therapy. Initial
responses to AEDs within 3 months and the presence or
absence of idiopathic epilepsy were the best predictors of
outcome. These data highlight the fact that childhood
epilepsy, often thought to be benign, can have significant
effects on mortality and require extended treatment.
Shinnar, et al (31) assessed the risk of multiple recurrences
after an initial seizure in 407 children followed for an average of 9.6 years from the time of their first seizure. A rising
risk of subsequent seizures over time was noted; the cumu-
lative risk of a second seizure was 29% through the first
year, 37% through the second year, 43% through the fifth
year, and 46% after ten years of follow-up. A second
seizure occurred in 182 children, while 72% of these children went on to have a third seizure, providing support to
the definition of epilepsy as the occurrence of more than
one unprovoked seizure. Further long-term assessment
studies of childhood epilepsy and the epilepsy syndromes of
childhood are crucial to identify the natural course and

prognoses of different seizure types and epileptic syndromes, as well as the effectiveness of different treatment
options.

Varying rates of epilepsy and of co-morbidity have been
found, depending on the geographical area and the population of children under study. Murphy and colleagues (25)
identified varying prevalence rates among children of different racial groups in Atlanta; prevalence among Caucasian
children was 5.7/1000 as compared to 6.4/1000 among
African Americans. The same study found increased risks
of co-morbidities, primarily in the form of mental retardation and cerebral palsy. It also revealed a sharp contrast
between childhood epilepsy with a good prognosis for even-
tual remission and epilepsy which does not remit and
which carries with it a substantial risk of death. Mortality
levels are raised in children with epilepsy, even among children with "epilepsy only," with marked increases seen in
children with epilepsy and other developmental disabilities
(32). A study of infantile spasms in Atlanta's children documented a poor prognosis for these youngsters: 94% had
active epilepsy at age 10 and 15% died before age 11 (33).
While these snapshots of specific prevalence rates are
informative, active surveillance of new cases sustained over
years is clearly needed, particularly of homogeneous epilepsy syndromes that may lead to identification of EEG, clinical and genetic markers, specific outcomes in sub-groups,
identification of trends or clusters, and more information
about the etiologic factors involved. EEG lab-based surveillance is one approach that should be considered.

Seizures in the elderly

The incidence of epilepsy rises sharply after age 60,
increasing to 139/100,000/year for people at 75 years of
age (2). This observation is particularly significant because
people aged 60 or older comprise the fastest growing segment of the U.S. population. Age affects multiple characteristics of epilepsy, including incidence, etiology, clinical
manifestations, treatment, AED pharmacology, efficacy,
side effects and prognosis (34). The recently completed
long-term multi-center VA study #428 evaluated epilepsy
characteristics and treatment in 594 elderly people (over 60
years of age) with seizures (35). The most common cause
of seizures in this group of elderly people, and in previous
studies, was cerebrovascular disease, yet no systems exist to
track and evaluate people post-stroke for the occurrence of
seizures or to test strategies to lessen the risk of developing
epilepsy.

Co-morbidities in older persons also are high, possibly
contributing to risks of seizures. The VA Cooperative
Study reported the most common co-morbid conditions to
be risk factors or complications for cerebrovascular disease,
e.g. dyslipidemia (80%), hypertension (64.4%), stroke
(52.7%), cardiac disease (48.8%), dementia (35.5%), and
diabetes (26.6%). The use of concurrent medications is

also high in older persons with seizures, complicating treatment and increasing the risk of drug interaction (34). The impact of seizures on an elderly population may have a disproportionate effect on independence and quality of life, leading to institutional care that might otherwise not have had to take place. More knowledge of the prognosis and treatment of seizures in elderly people is clearly needed.

Epilepsy in minority populations

In her presentation to the workgroup, Dr. Hesdorffer noted that few studies have produced incidence and prevalence rates for minority populations. Those that have been done suggest that prevalence is from 1.5 to 2 fold higher in African Americans of all ages compared to the general population, and from 1.1 to 1.4 fold higher when only children are studied. One study of northern Manhattan populations suggests higher racial and ethnic disparities in the incidence of unprovoked seizures and epilepsy. Rates among blacks exceeded those of whites by factors of 6.4 and 2.4 for children and adults, respectively. Similarly, rates among Hispanics exceeded those among non-Hispanics by factors of 2.1 for children and 1.7 for adults. The black-white differences in incidence exceed those for prevalence, but data for incidence are sparse. Future studies are needed on incidence and prevalence from the same community, together with data on causes, seizure type and care seeking behavior among minorities that may aid in determining preventable causes and areas for intervention.

Mortality in epilepsy

Much more also needs to be known concerning mortality rates among people of all ages with epilepsy. As noted above, the rate is elevated among children, and especially among children with severe syndromes of childhood epilepsy, including the Lennox-Gastaut syndrome and infantile spasms. However, there is substantial evidence of higher than expected mortality rates among the general population of people with epilepsy. People with epilepsy have a mortality rate 2-3 times higher than the rest of the population. Risk of sudden death is 24 times that of the general population. Sudden unexpected death in epilepsy (SUDEP) is responsible for 2 to 17% of deaths of people with epilepsy (36).

Mortality in epilepsy can be related to several factors, including the etiology of the condition, seizure frequency and absence of control, seizure type, and co-existing neurological or other medical conditions (37, 38). Tonic-clonic seizures appear to carry more risk than other types; so does poor seizure control and the presence of other neurological impairments (39). Sudden unexplained death (SUDEP) appears to be due to an acute cardiac or pulmonary disturbance, but its cause is still not well understood (40, 41).

Mortality in epilepsy is clearly an under-appreciated, severe problem that should be more aggressively defined, tracked, and tackled. Incidence cohort studies are needed, though they will be difficult to obtain. More knowledge is needed about the causes of epilepsy-related mortality, its pathophysiology, and potential for prevention. Research findings must then be transmitted to the healthcare community with emphasis on prevention strategies to reduce these risks.

D. Priority Recommendations: Epidemiology and Surveillance

Based on the presentations given to the group, the comments of the reactors, and subsequent discussion of the issues described above, Workgroup B recommended the following to enhance the assessment of epilepsy as a public health priority:

1. **Develop and enhance the capacity and infrastructure for surveillance and epidemiological studies of persons with epilepsy.**
   a. Assess people with new-onset epilepsy to capture information on demographic characteristics, epilepsy types and syndromes, long-term effects of treatment, and impact of epilepsy as a co-morbid condition.
   b. Develop and incorporate mechanisms to ascertain level of seizure control and severity, including active seizures versus those in remission, and controlled versus refractory seizures, in the population affected by epilepsy.
   c. Improve understanding of the epidemiology, course, predictors, and outcomes for those who have good seizure control and who manage their seizures and lives successfully.
   d. Utilize measures of health-related quality of life (HRQOL) to monitor health status in the epilepsy population, track changes to better understand the natural history of epilepsy, and evaluate effectiveness of interventions from a personal health perspective.
   e. Identify risk factors for mortality and morbidity.
   f. Extend surveillance studies and epidemiological research to include special populations and groups, including geographic area residents, members of ethnic/racial groups, nursing home or extended care facility residents, veterans, and military personnel.
   g. Include the categories of: "seizures and seizure disorder/epilepsy" in all relevant public health data collection systems.

2. **Develop surveillance systems to examine health care utilization and resources for people with epilepsy.**
   a. Identify and track patterns of care, treatment, and

prevention efforts to detect disparities, barriers, gaps, and quality of epilepsy care.

   b. Incorporate mechanisms to identify types of providers of epilepsy care, delays in diagnosis and referrals to tertiary centers, accuracy of diagnosis, and use of non-medical care and community-based services.

3. **Expand research on mortality and epilepsy to increase understanding of the causes of death in epilepsy.**

   a. Identify risk factors for epilepsy-associated mortality, and distinguish between mortality associated with epilepsy and that attributable to underlying conditions (e.g. etiology, co-morbid conditions) using incident cohorts.

   b. Evaluate the pathophysiology of epilepsy-related death by increasing emphasis on basic science research into mortality and epilepsy.

   c. Create a database or registry of autopsy findings to facilitate the evaluation of death in epilepsy.

   d. Encourage the use of brain bank resources to facilitate the study of death in epilepsy.

4. **Expand research on co-morbid conditions and epilepsy.**

   a. Identify risk factors for morbidity, including co-morbid conditions associated with epilepsy (e.g. neurobehavioral conditions, reproductive disorders, bone health, injuries, health status).

   b. Include people with epilepsy and other medical conditions in incident cohorts to understand the scope, burden, and consequences of seizures in all groups.

   c. Develop mechanisms to determine the severity of epilepsy and disability in those with co-morbid conditions.

   d. Evaluate the risk of specific epilepsy treatments on neurobehavioral function, reproduction, and health status.

   e. Develop surveillance systems that can determine the prevalence of psychogenic non-epileptic seizures in people with seizures, epilepsy, and the general population.

Workgroup C
Self-Management

A. Charge

Workgroup C was charged to examine the following issues:

- What are the key elements of self-management and self-determination needed to create a model to work best for people with epilepsy?

- What are the key components/skills/strategies of successfully living with epilepsy?

- What do we have or need to measure the key elements of self-management and self-determination?

- How do we successfully promote self-management and self-determination?

B. Workgroup Speakers

Participants in this workgroup explored the assurance function of public health by examining self-management and self-determination models, programs, and research needs. The following background information was drawn from workgroup presentations and relevant sources.

Presenters
- Progress since *Living Well I*: Patricia Osborne Shafer, RN, MN, Beth Israel Deaconess Medical Center, Epilepsy Foundation Professional Advisory Board
- Self-determination models: Kate Rollason, The ARC of the United States
- Self-management models: Colleen DiIorio, RN, PhD, FAAN, Emory University School of Medicine
- Interventions & lessons learned: Mary Macleish, Epilepsy Foundation of Arizona

Reactors
- Lynda A. Anderson, PhD, Centers for Disease Control and Prevention
- Merle Buckland, Idaho State Independent Living Council
- Sally Crudder, Centers for Disease Control and Prevention
- Richard Kahn, PhD, American Diabetes Association

C. Background

Defining epilepsy self-management
   Self-management has been defined as both the process of managing epilepsy (42) and the steps or behaviors neces-

sary for people to control seizures and manage the effects of having a seizure disorder (43). Self-management does not imply that people manage their health independently, but that positive health outcomes are best achieved by an active partnership between the persons who live with the condition and their health care team.

Self-management programs have been developed and evaluated in other chronic disorders such as diabetes, arthritis, and asthma to facilitate and promote patient-provider partnerships. Epilepsy is also an excellent candidate for such an approach. People must learn how to manage chronic medications, identify factors that may affect seizure control, and modify lifestyle accordingly to help manage unpredictable seizures and prevent injury. Additionally, people must take steps to prevent or cope with the consequences of seizures on their health and daily life, while managing stigma and other barriers to independent living.

Until recently, epilepsy health education and care has focused primarily on medication compliance. Disease management programs have emphasized the need for education and frequent follow-up, but are primarily focused on medical outcomes from the provider perspective. Austin and colleagues (44) have developed a Chronic Care Model that emphasizes evidence-based, population-based, and patient-centered care and the need for both community and health care systems to work together to achieve desired outcomes. Nurses and behavioral scientists are exploring self-management models to identify critical factors that influence health behaviors and develop programs or strategies that improve these behaviors. Research is also contributing to the development of communication strategies and approaches that assist people in becoming more active partners and advocates in their care. The research is moving epilepsy self-management from a specific focus on medication compliance to promoting a truly comprehensive approach to patient-centered epilepsy care. However, little research has been done to develop and evaluate easy to use, reproducible programs that can be implemented and disseminated throughout the country.

Self-management models

A few models have identified core themes and components of self-management in epilepsy. Initially the health belief model was used to conceptualize self-management components and learning needs (45). This approach suggests that successful management of epilepsy depends on a person's knowledge, attitudes, skills and behaviors, and identified four major components of epilepsy management-seizures, medications, medical care and lifestyle concerns. A self-management summit of invited experts in 1996 began identifying critical themes that extended beyond educational needs and that incorporated guiding principles of self-determination. The importance of information/education, skill building, and support networks were emphasized

as critical aspects for all programs and audiences. Crucial to this approach is the recognition that the epilepsy experience is highly individualized and that management and educational outcomes should be tailored to the individual and his or her family and incorporate broader quality of life goals such as knowing how to care for self and seizures, coping well, being satisfied with life, and feeling independent and in charge (46).

Specific self-management tasks that people with epilepsy may face at different points in their lives have been conceptualized in a broader view—adding the dimensions of access to care and social relationships/community living, while expanding the tasks necessary to manage health care needs, personal care, and safety (47). Subsequent research has validated the importance of seizure and medication management (48), while a psychosocial model of epilepsy self-management, based on social-cognitive theory, has expanded these components to also incorporate stress, safety, and information management (49, 50).

Factors influencing health behaviors – what can be changed?

Self-efficacy, or confidence in one's abilities, has been demonstrated to play a significant role in understanding self-management behaviors in chronic disease (51), and is a significant predictor of successful medication management for people with epilepsy (52, 53). Likewise, support and expectations of family, friends, and powerful others such as health care professionals are often influential in determining the type of behaviors in which one chooses to engage (51). A person's self-concept and mood is thought to affect one's confidence, and thus their ability to manage their health. DiIorio's self-management model affirms these assumptions, suggesting that stigma and depression negatively influence self-efficacy and self-management behaviors (50). Higher perceived stigma in the child has also been associated with negative mood and attitudes, parental perceptions of stigma and young age, as well as less self-efficacy in managing seizures (54).

Other factors affecting medication management have been studied extensively with adherence being the most frequently cited area of concern. Noncompliance is commonly considered one of the most frequently noted precipitants of breakthrough seizures, with medication factors (e.g. increased number of drugs, frequent doses, and side effects) corresponding to more adherence problems (55, 56). In addition to self-efficacy and support noted previously, fear and attitudes towards epilepsy appear to influence successful medication management, all of which are potential areas for intervention (57). While medications are a mainstay of treatment for most people with seizures, modifying one's lifestyle to eliminate or avoid precipitants of seizures, cope with stress, and prevent injuries are crucial areas of patient education. However, recent work suggests that people may be less confident in their ability to make healthy lifestyle changes than to manage medications (58).

Research in other disorders such as diabetes suggests that patient-doctor communication and the impact on shared decision-making and control are important aspects to consider in the development of epilepsy self-management, particularly how the communication process evolves from asking questions to taking action (comments by reactor Lynda Anderson, PhD, *Living Well with Epilepsy II* conference, July 2003). The focus on individual needs and behaviors (comments by reactor Merle Buckland and by Workgroup C seeded committee member Thomas Creer, PhD, *Living Well with Epilepsy II* conference, July 2003) and the critical steps of assuming responsibility, accountability, and authority (comments by reactor Richard Kahn, PhD, *Living Well with Epilepsy II* conference, July 2003) must be central facets as well. However, people with epilepsy and family members often don't know what questions to ask or how to find quality health care that will enable them to be responsible and take action. The need to define quality care in epilepsy, from the patient perspective as well as from the provider perspective, is crucial if people are to feel empowered and get the care they need. Achieving these objectives will require people with epilepsy and providers to become more knowledgeable about epilepsy care and learn critical advocacy skills (comments by reactor Sally Crudder, *Living Well with Epilepsy II* conference, July 2003).

Merging themes of self-management and self-determination

One of the barriers to developing self-management programs is a disconnect between the terminology used by clinicians and researchers, and the real life needs and concerns of consumers. For example, the true meaning and relevance of the term 'self-management' to people with epilepsy remains uncertain. Common themes of self-management previously identified by consumers and professionals incorporated principles of self-determination, a concept used to describe living independent, self-directed lives. Recommended principles and guidelines of self-determination in epilepsy were first published in 1995 (59). Rollason (comments by reactor, *Living Well with Epilepsy II* conference, July 2003) suggested that self-determination principles for epilepsy emphasize the need for *freedom* (working together with health care professionals to make decisions and to live a meaningful life), *authority* (choices in independent living/staffing, and control over necessary resources), *support* (for reasonable accommodations and to organize resources meaningfully), *responsibility* (accept consequences of decisions and choices), and *confirmation* (importance of consumer role in designing service systems). These concepts extend the philosophy of self-determination—and of living with epilepsy—to a way of looking at

'who I am as a person with epilepsy and what my goals and needs are.' Self-management is then considered one aspect of self-determination. Both concepts emphasize the importance of consumer-centered and driven programs and goals. Within this model, success or failure is not judged solely in terms of having or not having seizures, but also on a person's quality of life and working towards an independent and self-directed life.

Self-management needs across the spectrum of epilepsy

One of the major barriers to educating people with epilepsy is their differing needs, particularly in relation to age at seizure onset and seizure severity. Most often, health care professionals decide what people should be taught and develop curricula accordingly, contrary to the consumer-driven approach. During this workgroup's deliberations, critical elements, skills, and strategies targeted to those with new-onset seizures, well-controlled epilepsy, and those with refractory seizures were identified. Meeting constraints prevented development of consensus on these areas, but clear patterns emerged that warrant further evaluation and testing by the public health and epilepsy communities and incorporation into easy to use programs.

- **For people with new-onset seizures:** Initial emphasis should be devoted to awareness of seizure symptoms and warning signs, knowing standards of good care, knowing how to access quality care and resources, and to developing coping skills to accept diagnosis and manage fears. Becoming informed and being aware of the range of experiences and treatment options, while having realistic expectations are critical to making informed decisions and learning to manage difficult situations. The impact and importance of disclosure early in the course of epilepsy should be considered, in an effort to help people develop a proactive attitude and self-advocacy skills. Support systems must recognize the value of peer-to-peer networks at this critical phase of learning about seizures.

- **For people with well-controlled epilepsy:** Programs should incorporate a 'working knowledge' of epilepsy, focusing on strategies to manage seizures and maintain health, with strategies to enhance self-efficacy, support networks, and family/community education. Skill development must also focus on risk assessment, effective communication, managing disclosure and stigma, self-advocacy, resiliency for relapse and recovery, and self-awareness.

- **For people with refractory or uncontrolled seizures:** Programs and materials must focus on empowerment, persistence, and seeing self as able, while staying informed, knowing standards of quality care, and knowing how to access resources. Coping skills expand to overcome barriers, display courage, recognize the time course for adapting and coping with seizures, and manage stress effectively. The importance of individualized goals for seizure control and quality of life are critical at this stage. Being supported and persistent in working towards 'no seizures and no side effects' will require more emphasis on communication, assertiveness, and advocacy skills. Managing consequences of epilepsy requires skills to cope with stigma, disclosure, and knowledge of legal rights and resources. Concerns and strategies pertinent to people with cognitive, emotional and behavioral disorders should be considered. Strong support systems are needed, as well as training on financial support and planning.

From theory to practice – the impact of education and support

Patient education and support programs are often conducted in epilepsy centers and community-based programs, yet there is little published literature on the impact of these programs on people with epilepsy and their families. Referral patterns to such programs differ markedly in the United States, possibly due to availability, accessibility, and lack of insurance coverage. As a result, too many people with epilepsy do not have access to necessary education and support programs, rehabilitation, or other non-medical services.

A review of community-based programs and materials that address aspects of self-management or self-determination reveal a wealth of information in different formats (e.g. print, video, internet), but little age-appropriate information, especially for young adolescents and seniors with seizures. Barriers to accessing information abound, most notably language barriers, cultural competence of information, literacy level, cost, availability, and lack of access to technology (comments by presenter Mary Macleish, *Living Well with Epilepsy II* conference, July 2003). The Epilepsy Foundation and its affiliates have been instrumental in fostering peer involvement and support networks, but similar barriers exist that affect their use, especially in underserved communities, and published outcomes are sparse. Many of these programs were also developed using self-help models that do not incorporate many of the desired self-management and self-determination principles. Materials to foster empowerment, right to choices, and access to care are available in printed and Internet forums, and, most notably, through the Epilepsy Foundation's "Speak Up, Speak Out" program, which teaches advocacy skills. Unfortunately, this program is geared to developing skills for legislative and system-wide changes, rather than teaching self-advocacy

strategies that can help people access needed resources or communicate more effectively. Programs designed to assist people with epilepsy to develop responsibility, make decisions and be independent are found primarily outside the medical community – in the independent living, educational, transitional, and self-determination fields. The public health community should work closely with the epilepsy community and other fields to test relevant programs and replicate best practices that would help young people with epilepsy develop into self-determined adults, capable of managing their health and independent living needs.

A review of intervention research in self-management has shown that cognitive behavioral therapy and counseling can have positive affects on one's psychological adjustment, quality of life, coping skills, sense of self-control, adherence, perceived control of seizures, and mood (comments by presenter Colleen DiIorio, *Living Well with Epilepsy II* conference, July 2003). Psychoeducational programs are implemented most often in epilepsy; unfortunately little research has been done to examine the most effective formats in relation to desired outcomes. For example, the Sepulveda education program has demonstrated improved knowledge of epilepsy, decreased fear of seizures, and safer medical self-management practices in one study evaluating program participants (60). A modular educational program (MOSES) has also shown improvements in knowledge and coping as well as improved seizure outcomes and greater satisfaction with treatment in people completing the educational program (61). One-on-one educational interventions by nurses, particularly with people who have newly diagnosed epilepsy in community settings, have been studied in the United Kingdom, suggesting benefits in many knowledge areas, including risk management and medication-taking strategies (62). Motivational interviewing has been tried in other disorders to guide clients in identifying barriers and benefits to change health behaviors (62). This technique incorporates the need to tailor strategies to patient goals and desire for change, and focuses on enhancing self-confidence.

Most of these programs attempt to transfer knowledge and change behaviors at some level, recognizing that personal responsibility and accountability must be part of the process. The role of the health care provider may vary from an active participant to a guide, advisor, and supporter. While these models and programs of self-care appear promising, they are still being developed and tested in epilepsy and thus are not yet widely available. Public health efforts must be directed to further development of programs that can address the educational, support, and self-efficacy needs of people with epilepsy, and disseminate best practices that support effective self-management. Additionally, the public health community must join together with consumers and the epilepsy community to foster change within health care systems so that patient-centered care is the standard and not the exception to epilepsy management.

D. Priority Recommendations: Self-Management

Participants in this workgroup formulated many recommendations on needs for research, policies, and programs to enhance self-management and self-determination as integral aspects of epilepsy care. Common constructs and concepts of both self-management and self-determination were deemed important to people with epilepsy, and a merging of the two constructs was encouraged. The following recommendations include priority areas consolidated under key themes:

1. **Enhance behavioral and social science research of people 'living with epilepsy' and self-management of epilepsy.**
   a. Encourage research to develop and refine tools and strategies for clinical and research use that measure self-management and self-determination as critical outcomes for people with epilepsy.
   b. Validate research on common self-management components and behaviors, and expand dimensions of self-management into measurable components for people of varying age, ethnicity, gender, and seizure severity.

2. **Facilitate the development and testing of self-management models that incorporate critical components for epilepsy.**
   a. Incorporate key concepts of self-determination and self-management in models of epilepsy self-management, with emphasis on individualized goals, responsibility, empowerment, self-efficacy, trust, respect, information, support, decision-making, and control.
   b. Ensure that models of epilepsy self-management are appropriately consumer-driven and focused.

3. **Ensure that programs recognize the spectrum of epilepsy and tailor content appropriately to people with well-controlled, refractory, and new-onset seizures.**
   a. Tailor content and strategies to people of different ages, gender, and ethnicity.
   b. Incorporate tools and strategies that enable people with epilepsy and families to assess and manage risks of seizures, treatments, and co-morbid conditions.
   c. Create model interventions that support self-management and self-determination in epilepsy and disseminate successful programs to health care professionals and epilepsy educators/advocates.

4. **Promote self-management and self-determination principles and programs in the care and services for people with epilepsy.**
   a. Foster systems of care that facilitate empowerment of people with epilepsy and informed decision-making.
   b. Encourage the adoption of approaches and attitudes that support epilepsy self-management and self-determination by health care providers, the public health community, and families and that are tailored to geographic areas and cultural differences.
   c. Encourage community-based non-profit epilepsy organizations to incorporate self-management and self-determination programs in their service delivery and develop mechanisms to assist in the evaluation of such programs.
   d. Incorporate the importance of self-management and self-determination in health communications and public health campaigns, emphasizing empowerment and working towards living well, while appreciating the burdens of epilepsy across the lifespan.

Workgroup D
Quality of Life – Impact and Outcomes

A. Charge

Workgroup D was charged to examine the following issues:

- How have health communications addressed the stigma of epilepsy since the first *Living Well with Epilepsy* conference, including campaign results, survey results, targeted audience, and insights gained?

- What are the issues that affect quality of life in people with epilepsy and to what extent does stigma impact quality of life? How does quality of life and stigma differ in relation to age, gender, and ethnicity?

- What are the gaps in knowledge concerning quality of life and how do the gaps translate into research priorities?

- To what extent can quality of life be addressed by public health initiatives? What is the appropriate role of federal agencies, state health departments, and non-governmental organizations in addressing stigma to improve quality of life? What quality of life issues and messages should receive priority?

B. Workgroup Speakers

In addressing these questions, Workgroup D discussions focused on epilepsy's personal and public health consequences, and what is currently known about the impact of these issues on quality of life and the role of stigma. The following background information is drawn from these presentations and related sources.

Presenters
- Personal health consequences: Selena Fuller, Epilepsy Foundation of Eastern Pennsylvania, and David Ficker, MD, University of Cincinnati Medical Center
- Mood disorders and quality of life: John J. Barry, MD, Stanford University Medical Center
- Impact on parenting: Lauren Beck, Parents Against Childhood Epilepsy
- Psychological issues and public health: Bruce P. Hermann, PhD, University of Wisconsin Medical Center
- Community resources: Darla Templeton, Epilepsy Foundation of the St. Louis Region
- Impact of stigma on adolescents and families: Joan K. Austin, RN, DNS, FAAN, Indiana University School of Nursing
- Overview of quality of life in epilepsy: Frank Gilliam, MD, MPH, Washington University School of Medicine

Reactors
- Sandra Cushner-Weinstein RPT, LCSW-C, Children's National Medical Center
- Rosemarie Kobau, MPH, Centers for Disease Control and Prevention
- Denise L. Pease, Epilepsy Foundation Board of Directors
- William H. Theodore, MD, National Institute of Neurological Disorders and Stroke

C. Background

For most people who have it, epilepsy is a chronic disease (63). Despite real advances, it remains a condition that affected individuals must manage along with all the other responsibilities, tasks, and activities of daily life. Epilepsy, especially seizures that do not respond to treatment, is under-recognized and treated, while the consequences – elevated mortality, injuries, risk of injury, and impaired quality of life – are serious, poorly appreciated, and add significantly to the burden of disease, a burden that has been likened to that produced by cancer, arthritis, or heart disease (29). Even patients with newly diagnosed, adult-onset epilepsy suffer almost immediate deterioration in quality of life; within three months of diagnosis, signifi-

cant differences in physical and emotional roles, as well as on energy level have been noted (64). While quality of life does not always correlate with seizure frequency (65), individuals with recurrent seizures are at increased risk for impaired health related quality of life (66). Some consequences of epilepsy are clearly related to seizure frequency: loss of driving privileges, for example, and, in many cases, unemployment. Loss of driving privileges may in turn contribute to loss of independence, inability to work, and financial insecurity. In a recent study, more than one third of adults with epilepsy were unemployed or unable to work, and significantly more lived in households with low income (30), compared to those without epilepsy. Side effects from medication have also been found to contribute substantially to impairment of quality of life and are a frequent concern of people with epilepsy (67, 68).

Fear of when and where the next seizure will occur and effects on cognition (including memory, attention and concentration) are also cited when people are asked to identify major problems associated with epilepsy (64). The impact of epilepsy on quality of life thus varies from one individual to another, depending upon the type and severity of epilepsy, the effects of its treatment, and other concomitant neurological and medical disorders. The influences of a supportive environment, including access to health care and psychological and social support, are also important factors. Furthermore, the quality of life of family members is also profoundly affected when a member of the family has epilepsy (69).

Psychiatric co-morbidity

Psychiatric co-morbidity is common in people with epilepsy (70). While the lifetime prevalence of depression in the general population is approximately 16.2%, its prevalence in people with epilepsy ranges from 8 to 48%, with a mean of 29% (71). Other mood disorders, such as bipolar disorder or unspecified mood disorder, have been diagnosed in 8.1% of people with epilepsy, which is higher than in those with chronic diseases such as diabetes or asthma. Although the incidence of psychogenic non-epileptic seizures is estimated at 2 to 33 per 100,000 in the general population, it is much higher in people with uncontrolled seizures. Psychogenic non-epileptic seizures have been reported in 10-45% of patients with refractory epilepsy (72, 73). Anxiety disorders are also common (74), affecting up to 52.3% of people with epilepsy. Anxiety and depression may also coexist in the same patient (75).

Although depression is almost twice as common in patients with epilepsy, patients with epilepsy remain untreated for depression (76). Clinical depression is significantly associated with poorer health related quality of life and greater seizure severity (77). In addition, suicide and suicide attempts range from 5 to 14.3% in people with epilepsy, which is 3 to 4 times greater than in the general population (78). In people with temporal lobe epilepsy (in which seizures take the form of episodes of uncontrolled automatic behavior), the risk of suicide and number of suicide attempts is even higher, ranging up to 25 times that of the general population (79).

Significant depression may also affect children with epilepsy (80). Children also are not being treated for mental health problems. A recent study showed that approximately 60% of children with epilepsy had a psychiatric diagnosis and greater than 60% had received no mental health treatment (81). Differentiating among depressive episodes as co-morbid conditions is often difficult. Mood changes and the occurrence of depression or anxiety may occur before, during, or after seizures and be manifestations of the ictal state. Further research is needed to better differentiate between mood states and seizures, as compared to distinct co-morbid conditions, and to improve treatment of these conditions.

Depression has been cited as the single most important predictor of health related quality of life (HRQOL), yet it often goes untreated or under-treated (80, 82). Research is needed to identify explanations for lack of treatment so interventions can be developed to address them. Possible reasons for under-treatment include generally unfounded concerns that antidepressants will make the seizures worse, neurologists' lack of adequate training in psychiatry, lack of reimbursement and access to providers of mental health care services, the belief that AEDs are already providing psychiatric as well as epilepsy treatment, and the fact that psychiatrists are not always interested in treating people with epilepsy. Emphasizing the high prevalence of psychiatric disorders in people with epilepsy also risks creating a 'double stigma.' However, valid and reliable psychometric tools exist to make the diagnosis of depression, and these should be tested in populations of people with epilepsy and more widely utilized in clinical practice (83). Despite the documented prevalence of psychiatric disorders in people with epilepsy, there have been no randomized placebo-controlled trials of the treatment of psychological problems in epilepsy. Studies are also lacking regarding memory rehabilitation and transition to employment – both key components of quality of life.

A means of assessing individual risk of developing the emotional, psychological, and social consequences of epilepsy should be more widely available. Research should be undertaken to develop a comprehensive risk assessment tool that could be used by professionals and consumers to better understand the risks and to guide them in making informed decisions regarding the care needs of individual patients. The unacceptable rate of suicide in the population of people with epilepsy is in itself a strong argument for greater attention to be paid to psychological and psychiatric co-morbidities of epilepsy and related opportunities for suicide prevention.

Cognitive issues

People with epilepsy may also suffer from cognitive dysfunction (such as difficulties with memory, attention, processing, concentration), which is also associated with a negative impact on quality of life (83, 84, 85). Many patients with epilepsy are unaware of their cognitive dysfunction, which hinders their adaptation to it. Factors with potential effects on cognition include the underlying disease, the effects of seizures, AED treatment, and other treatments such as brain surgery (86, 87). Some treatments may yield positive effects on cognition, such as vagus nerve stimulation (82); systematic studies are needed to identify which other types of treatment have positive or negative effects on cognition and to differentiate the effects of seizure from the specific effect of a treatment. Currently, there is no treatment available for cognitive dysfunction related to epilepsy and no public health focus on the problem. Both are needed.

Nor has prevention of cognitive difficulties received research attention. A review of research citations on epilepsy and memory from 1996 to 2003 show the research community with a much greater interest in identifying the problem (90 citations) than in determining how it might be addressed through rehabilitation (0 citations). Epilepsy and cognition difficulties have similarly attracted descriptive research (210 citations), and only 1 citation for cognitive rehabilitation in epilepsy. Similar results are found relative to learning disorders and interventions in mood disorders. There is a major need for research on prevention and effective interventions in all these areas.

Children's and parents' quality of life

The quality of life for many children with epilepsy is compromised. Studies show that having epilepsy in the early years affects many domains, and has a more severe effect than other chronic illnesses of early life (88, 89, 90). Quality of life is further diminished in the presence of frequent seizures and learning and related disabilities, but even intellectually normal children with epilepsy are more likely to have emotional, behavioral, and cognitive problems and to be less competent in socializing and school performance (91).

Parents of children with epilepsy have many worries (92) and face many problems associated with their children's epilepsy, such as delays to diagnosis, gaining access to specialists, dealing with restrictions at school, the presence of learning disabilities, and, too often, the impact of social rejection by other children and their parents. Parents may find themselves alone, forced to navigate complicated health care and social services systems without guidance. Parents must also come to terms with their children's condition while encouraging their child's efforts towards independence (93, 94). Parental anxiety in the face of all these stresses tends to further complicate the situation, for themselves and their children. When children of anxious parents have poorly controlled seizures and a co-morbid disability, the parents suffer a diminished quality of life (95). It is not uncommon for parents to cite ignorance and lack of resources as significant barriers to successful education of their children with epilepsy. Parents also desperately need information about how to facilitate the transition from school to employment, how to maximize their students' achievement, and how to improve their mood (96).

Stigma

Stigma remains a significant part of the burden of epilepsy and its effects on quality of life (97). It can affect people with epilepsy in several ways. It can be felt internally as feelings, thoughts and fears of being different and less worthy than others. It can be reflected interpersonally, when the actions of others lead to discrimination against people with epilepsy through exclusion and isolation. And it can be expressed at the institutional level, when insurance companies, hospitals, universities, and other institutions treat people with epilepsy in ways that are different, and negatively different, from treatment accorded to others.

Social stigma also affects perceptions of self and self-worth. Research has shown that adolescents with epilepsy feel different from their peers, fear being embarrassed if they should have a seizure in front of others, and are anxious and worried about others' opinions of them (98). In one survey, 69% of adolescents who did not have epilepsy said they would want their friends to tell them if those friends had the condition, yet only 46% said that they would tell if they had epilepsy themselves (7).

In efforts to decrease stigma and improve acceptance, educational campaigns tend to minimize the problems faced by people with seizures. Such efforts are well meaning in that they attempt to reduce the social distance between the person with epilepsy and other people; however, such messages in the public square are inconsistent with the real struggles that many people with epilepsy have with disabling co-morbidities such as cognitive and psychiatric problems, conditions that may affect their quality of life as much as or more than their seizures. It is important for the community as a whole to recognize the challenges that people face, to aid them in meeting these challenges whenever possible, and to advocate for research towards their resolution as well as for the elimination of seizures. Research is needed to develop and test interventions that will improve and/or prevent the development of internalized stigma in young people and to develop targeted communications strategies to reach those who generate interpersonal stigma.

Further research is desperately needed to better understand the burden of epilepsy and how to ameliorate it. However, to make positive changes, we must also better understand who succeeds in life and why. Understanding factors that may lead to successful life performance, (such

as the various roles of optimism-pessimism, self efficacy, and resilience) and how these may vary among cultures and social groups is critical to improve quality of life for people with epilepsy. Research to answer these questions should be incorporated into other epidemiological studies and clinical trials of people with epilepsy.

D. Priority Recommendations: Quality of Life – Impact and Outcomes

Many personal, social, and institutional consequences of epilepsy were explored leading to the priority recommendations outlined below:

1. **Improve the assessment and treatment of the mental health needs of people with epilepsy through professional education and research.**
   a. Establish standards of care for mental health issues in persons with epilepsy, including assessment and care in children.
   b. Increase the availability of mental health assessments and treatment at comprehensive epilepsy centers and within the public health system.
   c. Improve access to psychiatric care by building bridges between the mental health and epilepsy communities.

2. **Enhance resources and infrastructure necessary to improve access to social services and enhance quality of life of people with epilepsy.**
   a. Explore strategies to increase access to insurance coverage of mental health and social services for people with epilepsy.
   b. Train community advocates and specialists to bridge gaps affecting people with epilepsy among public health, community, and health care systems.
   c. Inform people of available resources, using a centralized database relevant to the needs of people with epilepsy, their families, and health care providers.
   d. Develop and test mechanisms to successfully connect people with resources in diverse geographical areas.
   e. Develop a database of existing literature that identifies problem areas and interventions to improve access to care and prevent secondary disability.
   f. Expand advocacy networks at community, state, and federal levels.
   g. Enhance efforts to develop partnerships among stakeholders in the neurological, disability, and public health communities.

3. **Improve understanding of risks and consequences of epilepsy and its treatment.**
   a. Educate health care providers, people with epilepsy and caregivers about known risks, co-morbidities, and consequences of epilepsy and treatment related effects.
   b. Develop a risk assessment tool that can be used by people with epilepsy, families, and health care professionals to identify risks and make informed decisions.

4. **Improve understanding of the impact of seizures and epilepsy on learning and cognition and ways to lessen and prevent these effects.**
   a. Define and determine the prevalence and implications of academic underachievement and learning disorders in children and adults with epilepsy.
   b. Support intervention studies on treatment of cognitive problems in children and adults with epilepsy.
   c. Convene stakeholders, including experts in cognition and rehabilitation, to design a randomized controlled trial to treat cognitive problems in children and adults with epilepsy.
   d. Develop evidence-based standards of care for children and adolescents with epilepsy and learning disabilities.
   e. Develop professional education programs and best practices that address neuro-developmental disorders affecting learning and cognition.

5. **Enhance efforts to combat stigma in epilepsy.**
   a. Develop and test research models related to personal perceptions of stigma.
   b. Evaluate the impact of patient empowerment and self-management models and programs on personal perceptions of stigma.
   c. Assess the impact of public education campaigns and specific messages on social stigma and apply the results to future campaigns.
   d. Identify barriers that reflect institutional stigma and develop action plan to eliminate these barriers.
   e. Develop mechanisms to track and address stigma in academic and workplace settings.

V. Summary

Epilepsy can have devastating effects on individuals and their families when not diagnosed or treated effectively. America has the capacity to prevent or mitigate many of the untoward social, cognitive, and emotional consequences of epilepsy. To accomplish this, however, seizures and their effects must be identified more accurately and tracked to better understand the scope, course, and outcomes of these disorders.

In 1994, the public health community began recognizing some of the unsolved issues and unmet needs of people with epilepsy, but much more still remains to be done. This second *Living Well with Epilepsy* conference was designed to chart a path for the public health community, and those who care for and about epilepsy, over the next five years. The public health assessment needs that have been identified will provide a more complete picture of what epilepsy is, and how it affects people of different ages and ethnic backgrounds. Policies and practices that will improve access to quality care, facilitate early recognition and treatment, and prevent secondary disability have been recommended to help people achieve seizure freedom and the quality of life they deserve. Our health care system, originally designed for care of people with acute care needs, must respond to view epilepsy as a chronic health problem. People with epilepsy need integrated health care services that are designed and based on ongoing public health assessments of need. These services must then be supported by a system that can assure timely access to the range of treatments and care demonstrated to be most effective. Such care should ensure the self-determination of those who are served. At the same time, more aggressive efforts to eliminate stigma are essential to remove epilepsy from the shadows, while its burdens are recognized, treated, and ultimately erased.

VI. REFERENCES

1. Begley CE, Famulari M, Annegers JF, et al. The cost of epilepsy in the United States: an estimate from population-based clinical and survey data. *Epilepsia.* 2000;41:342-351.

2. Hauser WA, Annegers JF, Rocca WA. Descriptive epidemiology of epilepsy: contributions of population-based studies from Rochester, Minnesota. *Mayo Clin Proc.* 1996;71:576-586.

3. Goffman E. *Stigma.* Englewood Cliffs, NJ: Prentice-Hall; 1963.

4. Kwan P, Brodie MJ. Early identification of refractory epilepsy. *N Engl J Med.* 2000;342:314-319.

5. Schlaug G, Patel M. Radiographic assessment of patients with epilepsy. In: Schachter S, Schomer D, eds. *The Comprehensive Evaluation and Treatment of Epilepsy: A Practical Guide.* San Diego, Calif: Academic Press Inc; 1997:37-60.

6. Management of newly diagnosed patients with epilepsy: a systematic review of the literature. Evidence Report/Technology Assessment Number 39, Publications No. 01-E038. Agency for Healthcare Research and Quality, February 2001.

7. Austin JK, Shafer PO, Deering JB. Epilepsy familiarity, knowledge, and perceptions of stigma: report from a survey of adolescents in the general population. *Epilepsy Behav.* 2002;3:368-75.

8. Kobau R, Price P. Knowledge of epilepsy and familiarity with this disorder in the U.S. population: results from the 2002 healthstyles survey. *Epilepsia.* 2003;44:1449-1454.

9. Morrell MJ, Sarto GE, Shafer PO, Borda EA, Herzog A, Callanan M. Health issues for women with epilepsy: a descriptive survey to assess knowledge and awareness among healthcare providers. *J Womens Health Gend Based Med.* 2000;9:959-965.

10. Spanaki MV, Shafer PO, Schachter SC, Epilepsy Foundation. Women and epilepsy initiative: knowledge among neurology residents about epilepsy-related issues in women: results of a survey. *Epilepsia.* 2003;44(suppl 9):292-293. Abstract.

11. Kwan P, Brodie MJ. Effectiveness of first antiepileptic drug. *Epilepsia.* 2001;42:1255-1260

12. Jeavons PM, Harper JR, Bower BD. Long term prognosis of infantile spasms: a follow-up report on 112 cases. *Dev Med Child Neurol.* 1970;12:413-421.

13. Devinsky O. Patients with refractory seizures. *N Engl J Med.* 1999;340:1565-1570.

14. Siddiqui A, Kerb R, Weale ME, et al. Association of multidrug resistance in epilepsy with a polymorphism in the drug-transporter gene ABCB1. *N Engl J Med.* 2003;348:1442-1448.

15. Kwan P, Brodie MJ. Refractory epilepsy: a progressive, intractable but preventable condition? *Seizure.* 2002;11:77-84.

16. Kwan P, Brodie MJ. Drug treatment of epilepsy: when does it fail and how to optimize its use? *CNS Spectr.* 2004;9:110-119.

17. Schachter SC. Treatment of seizures. In: Schachter SC, Shomer DL, eds. *The Comprehensive Evaluation and Treatment of Epilepsy: A Practical Guide.* San Diego, Calif: Academic Press; 1997:61-74.

18. French JA, Kanner AM, Bautista J, et al. Efficacy and tolerability of the new antiepileptic drugs, I: Treatment of new-onset epilepsy. Report of the TTA and QSS subcommittees of the American Academy of Neurology and the American Epilepsy Society. *Epilepsia.* 2004;45:401-409.

19. French JA, Kanner AM, Bautista J, et al. Efficacy and tolerability of the new antiepileptic drugs, II: Treatment of refractory epilepsy. Report of the TTA and QSS subcommittees of the American Academy of Neurology and the American Epilepsy Society. *Epilepsia.* 2004;45:410-423.

20. Wiebe S, Blume WT, Girvin JP, Eliasziw M. A randomized controlled trial of surgery for temporal lobe epilepsy. *N Engl J Med.* 2001;345:311-318.

21. Langfitt JT, Bronstein K. Use of surgical procedures in the treatment of epilepsy: intervention and outcomes. *Dis Manag.* 1999;5:23-40.

22. Optional purchasing specifications: epilepsy. GWUMC School of Public Health and Health Services. June 2002:1-19.

23. Gumnit RJ, Walczak TS, National Association of Epilepsy Centers. Guidelines for essential services, personnel, and facilities in specialized epilepsy centers in the United States. *Epilepsia.* 2001;42:804-814.

24. Berg AT, Langfitt J, Shinnar S, et al. How long does it take for partial epilepsy to become intractable? *Neurology.* 2003;60:186-190.

25. Murphy CC, Trevathan E, Yeargin-Allsopp M. The prevalence of epilepsy in ten year old children: results from the Atlanta developmental disabilities study. *Epilepsia.* 1995;36:866-872.

26. Centers for Disease Control and Prevention. Health-related quality of life among persons with epilepsy – Texas 1998. *MMWR.* 2001;50:24-26.

27. Kobau R, DiIorio CA, Price PH, et al. Prevalence of epilepsy and health status of adults with epilepsy in Georgia and Tennessee: Behavioral Risk Factor Surveillance System, 2002. *Epilepsy Behav.* 2004;5:358-366.

28. Bazil C, Kothari M, Luciano D, et al. Provocation of nonepileptic seizures by suggestion in a general seizure population. *Epilepsia.* 1994;35:768-770.

29. Prueter C, Schultz-Venrath U, Rimpau W. Dissociative and associated psychopathological symptoms in patients with epilepsy, pseudoseizures, and both seizure forms. *Epilepsia.* 2002;43:188-192.

30. Sillanpaa M, Jalava M, Kaleva O, Shinnar S. Long-term prognosis of seizures with onset in childhood. *N Engl J Med.* 1998;338:1916-1918.

31. Shinnar S, Berg AT, O'Dell C, Newstein D, Moshe SL, Hauser WA. Predictors of multiple seizures in a cohort of children prospectively followed from the time of their first unprovoked seizure. *Ann Neurol.* 2000;48:140-147.

32. Decoufle P, Autry A. Increased mortality in children and adolescents with developmental disabilities. *Pediatr Perinat Epidemiol.* 2002;16:375-382.

33. Travathen E, Murphy CC, Yeargin-Allsopp M. The descriptive epidemiology of infantile spasms among Atlanta children. *Epilepsia.* 1999;40:748-751.

34. Ramsay RE, Pryor F. Epilepsy in the elderly. *Neurology.* 2000;55(suppl 1):S9-S14.

35. Ramsay RE, Rowan AJ, Pryor F. Treatment of seizures in the elderly: final analysis from DVA cooperative study 428. *Epilepsia.* 2003;44(suppl 9):170. Abstract.

36. Ficker D. Sudden unexplained death and injury in epilepsy. *Epilepsia.* 2000;41(suppl 2):S7-S12.

37. Cockerell OC, Johnson AL, Sander JW, Hart YM, Goodridge DM, Shorvon SD. *Lancet.* 1994;344:918-921.

38. Forsgren L, Edvinsson SO, Nystrom L, Blomquist HK. Influence of epilepsy on mortality in mental retardation: an epidemiologic study. *Epilepsia.* 1996;37:956-963.

39. Sperling MR, Feldman H, Kinman J, et al. Seizure control and mortality in epilepsy. *Ann Neurol.* 1999;46:45-50.

40. Schraeder PL, Lathers CM. Paroxysmal autonomic dysfunction, epileptogenic activity and sudden death. *Epilepsy Res.* 1989;3:55-62.

41. Blum AS, Ives JR, Goldberger AL, et al. Oxygen desaturations triggered by partial seizures: implications for cardiopulmonary instability in epilepsy. *Epilepsia.* 2000;41:536-541.

42. Shafer PO, Santilli N. Counseling parents and prospective parents with epilepsy. *Clin Nurs Pract Epilepsy.* 1996;3:10.

43. DiIorio C. Epilepsy self-management. In: Gochman DS, ed. *Handbook of Health Behavior Research II: Provider Determinants.* New York, NY: Plenum Press; 1997:213-230.

44. Austin B, Wagner E, Hindmarsh M, Davis C. Elements of effective chronic care: a model for optimizing outcomes for the chronically ill. *Epilepsy Behav.* 2000;1:S15-S20.

45. Shope JT. Educating patients and families to manage a seizure disorder successfully. In: Santilli N, ed. *Managing Seizure Disorders: A Handbook for Health Care Professionals.* Philadelphia, Pa: Lippincott-Raven Publishers; 1996:123-134.

46. Santilli N, Shafer PO. Health education and epilepsy self-management: summary report of conference proceedings, 1996.

47. Shafer PO. Epilepsy and seizures: advances in seizure assessment, treatment, and self-management: neuroscience nursing for a new millennium. *Nurs Clin North Am.* 1999;34:743-759.

48. Buelow JM. Epilepsy management issues and techniques. *J Neurosci Nurs.* 2001;33:260-269.

49. DiIorio C, Hennessy M, Manteuffel B. Epilepsy self-management: a test of a theoretical model. *Nurs Res.* 1996;45:211-217.

50. DiIorio C, Shafer P, Letz R, Henry T, Schomer D, Yeager K. The association of stigma with self-management and perceptions of health care among adults with epilepsy. *Epilepsy Behav.* 2003;4:259-267.

51. Bandura A. *Self-efficacy: the exercise of control.* New York, NY: W.H. Freeman and Co.; 1997.

52. DiIorio C, Faherty B, Manteuffel B. Self-efficacy and social support in self-management of epilepsy. *West J Nurs Res.* 1992;14:292-303.

53. DiIorio C, Faherty B, Manteuffel B. Epilepsy self-management: partial replication and extension. *Res Nurs Health.* 1994;17:167-174.

54. Austin JK, MacLeod J, Dunn DW, Shen J, Perkins SM. Measuring stigma in children with epilepsy and their parents: instrument development and testing. *Epilepsy Behav.* 2004;5:472-482.

55. Cramer J, Vachon L, Desforges C, Sussman NM. Dose frequency and dose interval compliance with multiple antiepileptic medications during a controlled clinical trial. *Epilepsia.* 1995;36:1111-1117.

56. Buck D, Jacoby A, Baker GA, Chadwick DW. Factors influencing compliance with antiepileptic drug regimes. *Seizure.* 1997;6:87-93.

57. Kyngas H. Compliance with health regimens of adolescents with epilepsy. *Seizure.* 2000;9:598-604.

58. Kobau R, DiIorio C. Epilepsy self-management: a comparison of self-efficacy and outcome expectancy for medication adherence and lifestyle behaviors among people with epilepsy. *Epilepsy Behav.* 2003;4:217-225.

59. Troxell J, Parks-Trusz S, Jepsen L. Independence and self-determination for persons with epilepsy: proceedings of the educational seminar on independence and self-determination. International Bureau for Epilepsy, the Netherlands: 1996.

60. Helgeson DC, Mittan R, Tan SY, Chayasirisobhon S. Sepulveda epilepsy education: the efficacy of a psychoeducational treatment program in treating medical and psychosocial aspects of epilepsy. *Epilepsia.* 1990;31:75-82.

61. May TW, Pfafflin M. The efficacy of an educational treatment program for patients with epilepsy (MOSES): results of a controlled, randomized study: modular service package epilepsy. *Epilepsia.* 2002;43:539-549.

62. Ridsdale L, Kwan I, Morgan M. How can a nurse intervention help people with newly diagnosed epilepsy? a qualitative study of patient views. *Seizure.* 2003;12:69-73.

63. Santilli N, Kessler BL, Schmidt WT. Quality of life in epilepsy: perspectives of patients. In: Trimble MR, Dodson WE, eds. *Epilepsy and Quality of Life.* New York, NY: Raven Press; 1994: 2.

64. Hughes C, Ficker D. Comparison of health related quality of life in newly diagnosed seizures with population norms. *Epilepsia.* 2003;44 (suppl 9):183-4. Abstract.

65. Arnston P, Droge D, Norton R, Murray E. The perceived psychosocial consequences of having epilepsy. In: Whitman S, Hermann B, eds. *Psychopathology in epilepsy: social dimensions.* New York, NY: Oxford University Press; 1986: 143-161.

66. Leidy NK, Elixhasuer A, Vickrey B, et al. Seizure frequency and health-related quality of life of adults with epilepsy. *Neurology.* 1999;53:162-166.

67. Ficker D, Hughes C, Shukla R, Privitera MD. Determinants of health-related quality of life in newly diagnosed seizures. *Epilepsia.* 2003;44(suppl 9):182. Abstract.

68. Fisher RS, Vickrey BG, Gibson P, et al. The impact of epilepsy from the patient's perspective II: views about therapy and health care. *Epilepsy Res.* 2000;41:53-61.

69. Thompson PJ, Upton D. Quality of life in family members of persons with epilepsy. In: Trimble MR, Dodson WE, eds. *Epilepsy and Quality of Life.* New York, NY: Raven Press;1994:19-31.

70. Hermann BP, Seidenberg M, Bell B. Psychiatric co-morbidity in chronic epilepsy: identification, consequences and treatment of major depression. *Epilepsia.* 2000;41(suppl 2):S31-S41.

71. Hermann BP, Blum D, Reed M, Metz A. Prevalence of major affective disorders and manic/hypomanic symptoms in persons with epilepsy: a community survey. *Neurology.* 2002;58(suppl): A174.

72. Bazil, C, Kothari M, Luciano D, et al. Provocation of nonepileptic seizures by suggestion in a general seizure population. *Epilepsia.* 1994;35:768-770.

73. Rowan AJ, Gates JR, eds. *Non-epileptic seizures.* Boston, MA: Butterworth-Heinemann; 1993:275-283.

74. Gupta AK, Ettinger AB, Weisbrot DM. Psychiatric comorbidities in epilepsy. In: Ettinger AB, Devinsky O, eds. *Managing Epilepsy and Co-existing Disorders.* Boston, Mass: Butterworth-Heinemann; 2002:343-387.

75. Victoroff J. DSM-III-R psychiatric diagnoses in candidates for epilepsy surgery: lifetime prevalence. *Neuropsychiatry Neuropsychol Behav Neurol.* 1994;7:87-97.

76. Wiegartz P, Seidenberg M, Woodard A, Gidal B, Hermann B. Co-morbid psychiatric disorder in chronic epilepsy: recognition and etiology of depression. *Neurology.* 1999;53(suppl 2):S3-S8.

77. Cramer JA, Blum D, Reed M, et al. The influence of co-morbid depression on quality of life for people with epilepsy. *Epilepsy Behav.* 2003;4:515-521.

78. Jones JE, Hermann BP, Barry JJ, Gilliam FG, Kanner AM, Meador KJ. Rates and risk factors for suicidal ideation, and suicide attempts in chronic epilepsy. *Epilepsy Behav.* 2003:4(suppl 3):S31-S38.

79. Barraclough BM. The suicide rate of epilepsy. *Acta Psychiatr Scand.* 1987;76:339-345.

80. Ettinger A, Weisbrot DM, Nolan EE, et al. Symptoms of depression and anxiety in pediatric epilepsy patients. *Epilepsia.* 1998;39:595-599.

81. Ott D, Siddarth P, Gurbani S, Koh S, Tourney A, Shields, WD, et al. Behavioral disorders in pediatric epilepsy: unmet psychiatric need. *Epilepsia.* 2003;44:591-597.

82. Clark KB, Naritoku DK, Smith DC, et al. Enhanced recognition memory following vagus nerve stimulation in human subjects. *Nature Neurosci.* 1999;2:94-98.

83. Sanchez-Carpintero, R, Neville, B. Attentional ability in children with epilepsy. *Epilepsia.* 2003;44:1340-1349.

84. Kalviainen R, Aikia M, Helkala EL, et al. Memory and attention in newly diagnosed epileptic seizure disorder. *Seizure.* 1992;1:255-262.

85. Piccirilli M, D'Alaessandro P, Sciarma T, et al. Attention problems in epilepsy: possible significance of the epileptogenic focus. *Epilepsia.* 1994;35:1091-1096.

86. Motemedi G, Meador K. Epilepsy and cognition. *Epilepsy Behav.* 2003;4:s25-s38

87. Halmstaedter C. Neurological aspects of epilepsy surgery. *Epilepsy Behav.* 2004;5:s45-s55.

88. Austin JK, Huster GA, Dunn DW, et al. Adolescents with active or inactive epilepsy or asthma: a comparison of quality of life. *Epilepsia.* 1996;37:1228-1238.

89. Hoare, P, Mann H. Self-esteem and behavioral adjustment in children with epilepsy and children with diabetes. *J Psychosom Res.* 1994;38:859-869.

90. Devinsky O, Westbrook L, Cramer J, et al. Risk factors for poor health-related quality of life in adolescents with epilepsy. *Epilepsia.* 1999;40:2715-2720.

91. Sabaz M, Cairns DR, Lawson JA, et al. The health-related quality of life of children with refractory epilepsy: a comparison of those with and without intellectual disability. *Epilepsia.* 2001;42:621-628.

92. Austin JK, Oruche UM, Dunn DW, Levstek DA. New-onset childhood seizures: Parents' concerns and needs. *Clin Nurs Pract Epilepsy.* 1995;2:8-10.

93. Austin JK. Assessment of coping mechanisms used by parents and children with chronic illness. *Am J Matern Child Nurs.* 1990;15:98-102.

94. Austin JK. A model of family adaptation to new-onset childhood epilepsy. *J Neurosci Nurs.* 1996;28:82-92.

95. Williams J, Steel C, Sharp GB, et al. Parental anxiety and quality of life in children with epilepsy. *Epilepsy Behav.* 2003;4:483-486.

96. Shore C, Austin JK, Musick B, Dunn D, McBride A, Creasy K. Psychosocial care needs of parents of children with new-onset seizures. *J Neurosci Nurs.* 1998;30:169-174.

97. Jacoby A. Stigma. Epilepsy and quality of life. *Epilepsy Behav.* 2002;3:S10-S20.

98. Austin JK. Concerns and fears of children with seizures. *Clin Nurs Pract Epilepsy.* 1993;1:4-6.

VII. APPENDICES

APPENDIX A:
Complete Listing of Recommendations for the *Living Well with Epilepsy II* Conference

A. Early Recognition, Diagnosis and Treatment

Priority Recommendations

1. **Support research to evaluate existing best practices and standards of care for persons with epilepsy.**
   a. Support and encourage health services and outcomes research to evaluate the impact of various levels and types of epilepsy care, including critical non-physician services and education.
   b. Support a randomized trial of 'customary care' versus early referral to specialized care.
   c. Support clinical research to evaluate the long-term benefits, risks, and costs of all treatment alternatives for seizures and epilepsy, including the risks and benefits of treatments on learning, cognition, and health-related quality of life (HRQOL) *(also identified in C and D)*.

2. **Improve understanding of seizures and epilepsy and best practices for epilepsy management, including referral to tertiary level of care, particularly for primary care providers.**
   a. Develop consensus on definitions and indicators of quality care for epilepsy *(also identified in C)*.
   b. Enhance communication and dissemination of standards of care and best practices among health care professionals, the public health community, health plans/insurers, people with epilepsy, and families.
   c. Undertake a "living with epilepsy" campaign to empower people with epilepsy and professionals to work aggressively towards the goals of 'no seizures and no side effects'. Incorporate information on patient and family expectations and rights, guidelines and indicators of quality care, how to access care, and community resources for epilepsy education and support *(also identified in C and D)*.

3. **Improve early recognition and timely diagnosis of seizures and epilepsy, including rare forms of seizures.**
   a. Develop and implement public awareness and education campaigns on seizure recognition and diagnosis targeted to first responders, school personnel, and health care professionals.
   b. Enhance dissemination of educational materials to emergency rooms, diagnostic laboratories, mental health clinics and primary health care sites.
   c. Enhance efforts to survey the general public's awareness, attitudes, and knowledge of epilepsy, including perceived barriers to seizure recognition and diagnosis *(also identified in C and D)*.

4. **Improve access to optimal care for persons with epilepsy.**
   a. Conduct demonstration projects to improve access to care in both urban and rural areas and among diverse population groups *(also identified in C)*.
   b. Replicate successful community programs that promote early recognition, timely diagnosis, and access to appropriate care, particularly to underserved geographical areas and groups.
   c. Improve the availability of specialized comprehensive care nationwide and encourage practices and systems that support comprehensive epilepsy care.

5. **Improve recognition and use of appropriate seizure first aid** *(also identified in C)*.
   a. Develop consensus criteria on the warning signs of seizures and epilepsy.
   b. Develop and implement educational programs for the general public on the warning signs of seizures in order to enhance early recognition.
   c. Support the development and dissemination of school-based epilepsy curricula to enhance seizure recognition and first aid.
   d. Promote universal teaching of appropriate seizure first aid as a component of standard first aid curriculums for schools and the general public *(also identified in C)*.

6. **Enhance understanding of mortality in epilepsy among all audiences** *(also identified in B)*.
   a. Develop educational materials and programs on death in epilepsy and preventable causes for professional and lay audiences.
   b. Incorporate the relationship of mortality to seizure severity and control in educational materials.
   c. Evaluate best practices to reduce mortality, particularly the impact of early intervention.
   d. Create support systems and resources for families and caregivers to assist in coping with epilepsy-related death.

7. **Enhance professional education on seizures and epilepsy, particularly to primary care providers and health care professionals in training.**
   a. Collaborate with medical schools, universities, and professional organizations to develop strategies and policies for recruitment, training and retention of epileptologists and other epilepsy specialists.
   b. Utilize problem-oriented case vignettes to target areas of high need (i.e. evaluation of new-onset seizures, pregnancy counseling, age and gender-specific issues related to epilepsy, educational and job related counseling, and when to discontinue medications) in professional educational programs for primary care providers and neurologists.

8. **Improve systems of care for people with epilepsy.**
   a. Test new strategies to improve access to care (e.g. yearly specialty consultations, use of telemedicine) and enhance working relationships between community-based providers and epilepsy specialists.
   b. Support the development of public health clinics specializing in epilepsy to improve access to care and prevent secondary disability for people with seizures in underserved areas.

9. **Expand health services research to improve access to care.**
   a. Encourage research to identify barriers to accessing care in underserved communities and the impact of literacy, cultural differences, and stigma. Test strategies to eliminate barriers and improve access to care in these communities.
   b. Define criteria and specifications of care for special populations of people with epilepsy [e.g. specific age groups (women, elderly, children, veterans), people who are developmentally delayed, people with co-morbidities].
   c. Encourage research to understand the educational needs and knowledge of epilepsy of health care providers at different levels of care.

B. Epidemiology And Surveillance

Priority Recommendations

1. **Develop and enhance the capacity and infrastructure for surveillance and epidemiologic studies of persons with epilepsy.**
   a. Assess people with new-onset epilepsy to capture information on demographic characteristics, epilepsy types and syndromes, long-term effects of treat-

ment, and impact of epilepsy as a co-morbid condition.
   b. Develop and incorporate mechanisms to ascertain levels of seizure control and severity, including active seizures versus those in remission, and controlled versus refractory seizures in the population affected by epilepsy.
   c. Improve understanding of the epidemiology, course, predictors, and outcomes for those who have good seizure control and those who manage their seizures and lives successfully *(also identified in A and C)*.
   d. Utilize measures of health-related quality of life (HRQOL) to monitor health status in the epilepsy population, track changes to better understand the natural history of epilepsy, and evaluate effectiveness of interventions from a personal health perspective *(also identified in D)*.
   e. Identify risk factors for mortality and morbidity *(also identified in D)*.
   f. Extend surveillance studies and epidemiologic research to include special populations and groups, including geographic area residents, members of ethnic/racial groups, nursing home or extended care facility residents, veterans, and military personnel.
   g. Include the categories of: "seizures, and seizure disorder/epilepsy" in all relevant public health data collection systems.

2. **Develop surveillance systems to examine health care utilization and resources for people with epilepsy.**
   a. Identify and track patterns of care, treatment and prevention efforts to detect disparities, barriers, gaps, and quality of epilepsy care *(also identified in A)*.
   b. Incorporate mechanisms to identify types of providers of epilepsy care, delays in diagnosis and referrals to tertiary centers, accuracy of diagnosis, and use of non-medical care and community-based services *(also identified in A)*.

3. **Expand research on mortality and epilepsy to increase understanding of the causes of death in epilepsy.**
   a. Identify risk factors for epilepsy-associated mortality, and distinguish between mortality associated with epilepsy and that attributable to underlying conditions (e.g. etiology, comorbid conditions) using incident cohorts.
   b. Evaluate the pathophysiology of epilepsy-related death by increasing emphasis on basic science research into mortality and epilepsy.
   c. Create a database or registry of autopsy findings to

facilitate the evaluation of death in epilepsy.

    d. Encourage the use of brain bank resources to facilitate the study of death in epilepsy.

4. **Expand research on co-morbid conditions and epilepsy** *(also identified in D)*.

    a. Identify risk factors for morbidity, including co-morbid conditions associated with epilepsy (e.g. neurobehavioral conditions, reproductive disorders, bone health, injuries, health status) *(also identified in D)*.

    b. Include people with epilepsy and other medical conditions in incident cohorts to understand the scope, burden and consequences of seizures in all groups *(also identified in D)*.

    c. Develop mechanisms to determine the severity of epilepsy and disability in those with co-morbid conditions.

    d. Evaluate the risk of specific epilepsy treatments on neurobehavioral function, reproduction, and health status *(also identified in A, C, and D)*.

    e. Develop surveillance systems that can determine the prevalence of psychogenic non-epileptic seizures in people with seizures, epilepsy and the general population *(also identified in A)*.

C. Self-Management

Priority Recommendations

1. **Enhance behavioral and social science research of people 'living with epilepsy' and self-management of epilepsy.**

    a. Encourage research to develop and refine tools and strategies for clinical and research use that measure self-management and self-determination as critical outcomes for people with epilepsy.

    b. Validate research on common self-management components and behaviors, and expand dimensions of self-management into measurable components for people of varying age, ethnicity, gender, and seizure severity.

2. **Facilitate the development and testing of self-management models that incorporate critical components for epilepsy.**

    a. Incorporate key concepts of self-determination and self-management in models of epilepsy self-management, with emphasis on individualized goals, responsibility, empowerment, self-efficacy, trust, respect, information, support, decision-making, and control.

    b. Ensure that models of epilepsy self-management

are appropriately consumer-driven and focused.

3. **Ensure that programs recognize the spectrum of epilepsy and tailor content appropriately to people with well-controlled, refractory, and new-onset seizures.**

    a. Tailor content and strategies to people of different ages, gender and ethnicity.

    b. Incorporate tools and strategies that enable people with epilepsy and families to assess and manage risks of seizures, treatments, and co-morbid conditions *(also identified in D)*.

    c. Create model interventions that support self-management and self-determination in epilepsy and disseminate successful programs to health care professionals and epilepsy educators/advocates.

4. **Promote self-management and self-determination principles and programs in the care and services for people with epilepsy.**

    a. Foster systems of care that facilitate empowerment of people with epilepsy and informed decision-making *(also identified in D)*.

    b. Encourage the adoption of approaches and attitudes that support epilepsy self-management and self-determination by health care providers, the public health community, and families and that are tailored to geographic areas and cultural differences.

    c. Encourage community-based non-profit epilepsy organizations to incorporate self-management and self-determination programs in their service delivery and develop mechanisms to assist in the evaluation of such programs.

    d. Incorporate the importance of self-management and self-determination in health communications and public health campaigns, emphasizing empowerment and working towards living well, while appreciating the burdens of epilepsy across the lifespan.

Other Areas of Importance

5. **Focus epilepsy education programs on those components, skills and strategies that promote self-management and self-determination.**

    a. Develop strategies to assess readiness, desire and expectations to engage in self-management, using culturally appropriate tools that can be implemented in clinical and community-based settings.

    b. Develop strategies and programs to enhance self-efficacy, a critical factor affecting health behavior.

    c. Evaluate and disseminate best practices on shared

control and decision-making in chronic disease and their implications for epilepsy care.

   d. Incorporate and test critical elements of self-management common for all people with epilepsy.
- Being self-confident and seeing self as able (self-efficacy)
- Coping (e.g. acceptance, managing fears, denial of barriers, courage, assertive, self-aware, perceptions of control, resiliency)
- Establishing goals, expectations, outcomes
- Managing information and obtaining education on epilepsy and treatment
- Developing skills for planning, problem solving, decision-making
- Developing support systems
- Communicating effectively and assertively
- Accessing quality care for epilepsy and mental health
- Advocating for self
- Assessing risks
- Developing seizure action plans for seizure recognition and first aid
- Maintaining health – including needs unique to gender, age, developmental level, and seizure severity
- Managing treatment and side effects
- Managing lifestyle for seizures, safety, and stress management
- Identifying and managing consequences of epilepsy and co-morbid conditions
- Managing disclosure, discrimination, and stigma

6. Promote self-management and self-determination principles and practices in clinical and community care areas.

   a. Develop strategies to encourage public health agencies to have consumer-centered and driven policies, programs, and infrastructure to better meet the needs of people with epilepsy.

   b. Develop and disseminate templates of simple and practical educational strategies that can be adapted to target audience needs.

   c. Disseminate best practices that reinforce positive health behaviors, coping strategies, and realistic expectations and goals.

   d. Enhance access to reliable, culturally appropriate educational materials for people with diverse abilities on access to epilepsy care, mental health resources, and financial resources.

   e. Enhance web-based dissemination of information and services to people with epilepsy and caregivers.

   f. Improve awareness of Epilepsy Foundation resources in the general public, public health community, and underserved areas by expanding out-

reach and educational efforts.

   g. Encourage the continued efforts of the public health community and the Epilepsy Foundation to reach parents as a target audience for education.

   h. Educate health care professionals regarding their role in promoting and facilitating self-management.

   i. Expand awareness and use of positive role models and experiences, such as peer mentors, epilepsy camps, volunteer development, and support groups.

   j. Encourage further development of support networks that are flexible and tailored to persons with epilepsy and caregivers in different settings.

   k. Enhance collaboration with school nurses and develop new partnerships with other health care and community-based organizations to provide epilepsy education to children, elders, caregivers and educators.

   l. Work with private and public insurers and decision-makers for coverage and funding of epilepsy self-management education and specialized services.

7. Expand research on measuring outcomes of educational interventions and self-management programs.

   a. Develop tools to assess cultural differences and their impact on educational needs, self-management, outcome expectancies, and quality of life.

   b. Explore work in developmental disabilities and other chronic disorders to develop appropriate measures of self-determination, empowerment, resiliency, adaptability, provider trust, perceptions of control, and caregiver burden in epilepsy.

   c. Evaluate learning styles and timing of epilepsy education in relation to age of onset of epilepsy, seizure severity, and outcomes to determine optimal points for educational interventions.

   d. Expand research efforts to assess the impact of epilepsy education on behavior change, social attitudes, and health outcomes, and conduct comparative studies of different educational methods.

   e. Examine the impact of Epilepsy Foundation services on health outcomes, self-management behaviors, social attitudes, and supports.

   f. Modify existing seizure severity scales for wider application to people with epilepsy.

   g. Explore usefulness and feasibility of electronic monitoring and self-report as measures of medication adherence.

   h. Evaluate the impact of camp experiences on the confidence and independence of youth with epilepsy.

D. Quality Of Life – Impact and Outcomes

Priority Recommendations

1. **Improve the assessment and treatment of the mental health needs of people with epilepsy through professional education and research.**
   a. Establish standards of care for mental health issues in persons with epilepsy, including the assessment and care in children.
   b. Increase the availability of mental health assessments and treatment at comprehensive epilepsy centers and within the public health system.
   c. Improve access to psychiatric care by building bridges between the mental health and epilepsy communities.

2. **Enhance resources and infrastructure necessary to improve access to social services and enhance quality of life of people with epilepsy.**
   a. Explore strategies to increase access to insurance coverage of mental health and social services for people with epilepsy.
   b. Train community advocates and specialists to bridge gaps affecting people with epilepsy among public health, community and health care systems *(also identified in C)*.
   c. Inform people of available resources, using a centralized database relevant to the needs of people with epilepsy, their families, and health care providers *(also identified in C)*.
   d. Develop and test mechanisms to successfully connect people with resources in diverse geographical areas *(also identified in C)*.
   e. Develop a database of existing literature that identifies problem areas and interventions to improve access to care and prevent secondary disability *(also identified in A)*.
   f. Expand advocacy networks at community, state, and federal levels.
   g. Enhance efforts to develop partnerships among stakeholders in the neurological, disability, and public health communities.

3. **Improve understanding of risks and consequences of epilepsy and its treatment.**
   a. Educate health care providers, people with epilepsy and caregivers about known risks, co-morbidities, and consequences of epilepsy and treatment related effects.
   b. Develop a risk assessment tool that can be used by people with epilepsy, families, and health care professionals to identify risks and make informed decisions *(also identified in C)*.

4. **Improve understanding of the impact of seizures and epilepsy on learning and cognition and ways to lessen and prevent these effects.**
   a. Define and determine the prevalence and implications of academic underachievement and learning disorders in children and adults with epilepsy.
   b. Support intervention studies on treatment of cognitive problems in children and adults with epilepsy.
   c. Convene stakeholders, including experts in cognition and rehabilitation, to design a randomized controlled trial to treat cognitive problems in children and adults with epilepsy.
   d. Develop evidence-based standards of care for children and adolescents with epilepsy and learning disabilities.
   e. Develop professional education programs and best practices that address neuro-developmental disorders affecting learning and cognition.

5. **Enhance efforts to combat stigma in epilepsy.**
   a. Develop and test research models related to personal perceptions of stigma.
   b. Evaluate the impact of patient empowerment and self-management models and programs on personal perceptions of stigma.
   c. Assess the impact of public education campaigns and specific messages on social stigma and apply the results to future campaigns.
   d. Identify barriers that reflect institutional stigma and develop action plan to eliminate these barriers.
   e. Develop mechanisms to track and address stigma in academic and workplace settings.

Other Areas of Importance

6. **Assess and prioritize service needs of people with epilepsy and develop national needs-based standards for provision of services.**

7. **Improve the mental health and quality of life of persons with epilepsy and caregivers.**
   a. Encourage comprehensive care centers and community-based programs to incorporate quality of life measures in epilepsy care.
   b. Survey physicians and mental health providers on awareness of epilepsy and its effects on mental health.
   c. Develop professional education programs to improve recognition, diagnosis, and treatment of psychiatric disorders in people with seizures.
   d. Develop and distribute institution best practices for employment.
   e. Enhance and expand Epilepsy Month Awareness

activities, particularly to underserved areas.

   f.   Strengthen anti-discrimination measures and laws.

   g.   Partner with disability and educational groups to conduct a "Respect for Differences" campaign in schools to foster respect for children with disabilities, decrease stigma, and prevent bullying and school violence.

   h.   Conduct a "Breaking the Silence" campaign involving the 'silent successful' patients to combat stigma and improve public understanding.

8. Enhance research into consequences and co-morbidities associated with epilepsy.

   a.   Increase research on psychiatric co-morbidities in people with epilepsy of varying severity and in relation to gender and age.

   b.   Assess efficacy of psychosocial and psychopharmacologic interventions in treatment of depression associated with epilepsy.

   c.   Evaluate health-related quality of life for people with epilepsy who have received mental health care services.

   d.   Assess the extent and effect of stigma associated with a dual diagnosis of epilepsy and mental health issues.

   e.   Assess coping strategies and quality of life in seniors with seizures.

   f.   Evaluate the effectiveness of different mentoring models on quality of life.

APPENDIX B:
Activities Resulting from the 1997 *Living Well with Epilepsy* Conference

Public health programs and initiatives that have evolved from recommendations produced by the 1997 conference on epilepsy include the following resources and activities, either completed or in progress:

- Agency for Healthcare Research and Quality (AHRQ) Evidence Report, *Management of Newly Diagnosed Patients with Epilepsy: A Systematic Review of the Literature.*

- AHRQ Evidence Report, *Management of Treatment-Resistant Epilepsy.*

- George Washington University Center for Health Services Research and Policy report, *Optional Purchasing Specifications For Services Related To Epilepsy.*

- Research examining health outcomes related to different levels of specialty care in pediatric patients with epilepsy.

- Programs and materials to help adolescents with epilepsy make informed decisions about issues of concern in their lives.

- Programs and materials to support parents of teens with epilepsy and help them assist their children in taking appropriate responsibility for managing their condition.

- *Epilepsy Self-Management Bibliography*, a collection of peer-reviewed articles that addresses the behavioral treatment and management of epilepsy.

- Epilepsy Education and Prevention Activities information, provided as part of the Combined Health Information Database.

- Studies implementing and evaluating self-management interventions in epilepsy.

- Analyses of national surveillance data sets and national mortality data to include trends in access to care, levels of care, and other demographic variables related to epilepsy.

- Studies to determine the prevalence of self-reported epilepsy in selected states using the Behavioral Risk Factor Surveillance System.

- Development of a method to identify cases of epilepsy in managed care organization populations and to enable studies of epilepsy incidence and prevalence using administrative health care data.

- Studies of cysticercosis in selected communities, in order to assess the associated risk of epilepsy and to develop more effective prevention programs.

- Development of an instrument to document public perceptions about people with epilepsy.

- Studies of the natural history and determinants of the occurrence, progression, and impact of epilepsy in older age.

- A study of the impact of transportation restrictions on the quality of life of people with epilepsy.

- Epidemiological studies of populations with epilepsy in northern Manhattan, New York City, and South Carolina.

- Multi-year public education campaigns to improve quality of life for adolescents and the elderly with epilepsy.

- Epilepsy curriculum development for students and school personnel.

- Collaborative project to examine issues and expectations for the role of states in addressing public health issues related to lower prevalence chronic conditions, using epilepsy as a model.

- Collaborative project with the National Conference of State Legislatures (NCSL) to educate state legislators about priority public health issues.

- Demonstration outreach to diverse populations, including local projects targeting African American, Amish, Arabic, Hispanic, and migrant worker populations.

APPENDIX C:
Conference Planning Committee, Speakers and Participants

Conference Co-Chairs

Gregory L. Barkley
Henry Ford Health System of Detroit
Epilepsy Foundation representative

Patricia Osborne Shafer
Beth Isreal Deaconess Medical Center
Epilepsy Foundation representative

Conference Planning Committee

Joan K. Austin
Indiana University
School of Medicine
American Epilepsy Society representative

Denise Cyzman
Michigan Department of
Community Health
Chronic Disease Directors representative

Donald J. Goodwin
South Carolina Department of
Health and Environmental Control
Chronic Disease Directors representative

Robert J. Gumnit
MINCEP Epilepsy Care
*National Associations of Epilepsy
Centers representative*

Margaret Jacobs
National Institute of Neurological
Disorders and Strokes

David Labiner
Arizona Comprehensive
Epilepsy Program
*National Association of Epilepsy
Centers representative*

Solomon L. Moshe
Albert Einstein College of Medicine
Yeshiva University
American Epilepsy Society representative

Patricia H. Price
Centers for Disease Control
and Prevention

Ellen Riker
MINCEP Epilepsy Care
*National Association of Epilepsy
Centers representative*

David Thurman
Centers for Disease Control
and Prevention

Fran Wheeler
National Association of
Chronic Disease Directors

Conference Summary

Gregory L. Barkley
Henry Ford Health System of Detroit

Deborah Carr
Epilepsy Foundation

Jody Kakacek
Epilepsy Foundation

Ann Scherer
Epilepsy Foundation

Patricia Osborne Shafer
Beth Isreal Deaconess Medical Center

Peter Van Haverbeke
Epilepsy Foundation

Andrew Wilner
Medical Communications

Opening Plenary Speakers

Cynthia Boddie-Willis
Massachusetts Division of
Community Health Promotion

Virginia S. Bales Harris
Centers for Disease Control
and Prevention

Deborah Jones-Saumty
American Indian Associates

Cynthia McCormick
National Institute of
Neurological Disorders and Stroke

Merle McPherson
Health Resources and
Services Administration

Solomon L. Moshe
Albert Einstein College of Medicine
Yeshiva University

Suzanne M. Smith
Centers for Disease Control
and Prevention

Linda K. Warner
Epilepsy Foundation
Board of Directors

Closing Remarks

Tony Coelho
Epilepsy Foundation
Board of Directors

Eric R. Hargis
Epilepsy Foundation

Workgroup A
Early Recognition, Diagnosis, and Treatment

Workgroup A Co-Chairs

Phillip Gattone
Epilepsy Foundation of
Greater Chicago

Martha J. Morrell
Columbia Presbyterian
Medical Center of New York

Workgroup A
Background Presenters

Susan Axelrod
Citizens United for
Research in Epilepsy

Santi K.M. Bhagat
Potomac, MD

John Booss
Veterans Administration Connecticut
Healthcare Systems

Susan Eik Filstead
Susan Eik Filstead Stroke and
Epilepsy Foundation, Inc.

Jacqueline A. French
The Neurological Institute at the
University of Pennsylvania

Gregory L. Holmes
Dartmouth-Hitchcock
Medical Center

Jeffrey Levi
George Washington University
Medical Center

Suzanne M. Smith
Centers for Disease Control
and Prevention

Workgroup A Members

Susan Axelrod
Citizens United for
Research in Epilepsy

Fay Bachman
Epilepsy Foundation of Arizona

Santi K.M. Bhagat
Potomac, MD

Jill Bonnett
Synergistic Healing

John Booss
Veterans Affairs Connecticut
Healthcare Systems

Marcia Buckminster
National Association of School Nurses

James C. Cloyd
University of Minnesota
College of Pharmacy

Jeffrey Cohen
Beth Israel Medical Cente
Singer Division

Guadalupe Corral-Leyv
Epilepsy Foundation of Los Angeles,
Orange, San Bernardino, and
Ventura Counties

Denise Cyzman
Michigan Department of
Community Health

Marc A. Dichter
Penn Epilepsy Center at the
University of Pennsylvania Hospital

Alan Ettinger
Long Island Jewish Medical Center

Susan Fahey
Parents Against Childhood Epilepsy

Susan Eik Filstead
Susan Eik Filstead Stroke and
Epilepsy Foundation, Inc.

Tracie J. Flourie
Del Mar, CA

Jacqueline A. French
University of Pennsylvania

Luukialuanna Garrison
Epilepsy Foundation of Los Angeles,
Orange, San Bernardino, and
Ventura Counties

Phillip Gattone
Epilepsy Foundation of
Greater Chicago

Arlene S. Gorelick
Epilepsy Foundation of Michigan

Robert J. Gumnit
MINCEP Epilepsy Care
National Association of
Epilepsy Centers

Virginia S. Bales Harris
Centers for Disease Control
and Prevention

Meenaxi Hiremath
National Institutes of Health

Susan Hoh
Mendon, NY

Gregory L. Holmes
Dartmouth-Hitchcock
Medical Center

Jill Hudson
Epilepsy Foundation

Marlene Jackovich
Epilepsy Foundation of Arizona

Margaret Jacobs
National Institute of
Neurological Disorders and Stroke

David Labiner
Arizona Comprehensive
Epilepsy Program

Mary Leveck
National Institute of Nursing Research

Jeffrey Levi
George Washington University
Medical Center

Gary Mathern
University of California
Los Angeles Medical Center

Christopher Maylahn
New York State
Department of Health

Debbie McGrath
Epilepsy Foundation of Kentuckiana

Colette Monier-Ridge
Shire US, Inc.

Linda Monroe
St. Luke's Regional Medical Center

Martha J. Morrell
Columbia Presbyterian
Medical Center of New York

Solomon L. Moshe
Albert Einstein College of Medicine
Yeshiva University

Christine L. O'Dell
Montefiore Medical Center

Judith O'Toole
Epilepsy Foundation

Lynne Panian
Epilepsy Foundation of
San Diego County

John Pellock
Virginia Commonwealth
University Healthsystem
Medical College of Virginia

Marty Puentis
Pharmaceuticals Health
Care Compliance

Frank J. Ritter
Comprehensive Epilepsy Program
of Minnesota

Judith Robinson
National Association of School Nurses

Tess Sierzant
Health East Care System
St. Joseph's Hospital
St. Paul, Minnesota

Brien J. Smith
Henry Ford Hospital

Suzanne M. Smith
Centers for Disease Control
and Prevention

David L. Snyder
Emergency Care Research Institute

Joan Spainhower
Florida Department of Health

Blanca Vazquez
New York University Medical Center

Julie Ward
Epilepsy Foundation

Heather Worland
Epilepsy Foundation of Kentuckiana

Workgroup B
Epidemiology and Surveillance

Workgroup B Co-Chair

W. Allen Hauser
Columbia University

Edwin Trevathan
Washington University
School of Medicine

**Workgroup B
Background Presenters**

Charles E. Begley
University of Texas
School of Public Health

Dale Hesdorffer
G.H. Sergievsky Center

R. Eugene Ramsay
University of Miami
School of Medicine

Michael R. Sperling
Thomas Jefferson University Hospital

Edwin Trevathan
Washington University
School of Medicine

Workgroup B Members

Anthony Anzalone
Cyberonics

Mary Alice Bare
Children's Hospital Medical Center
Cincinnati, Ohio

Ellen Becker
Epilepsy Foundation of
Southwestern Illinois

Charles E. Begley
University of Texas
School of Public Health

Suzanne C. Berry
American Epilepsy Society

Peter Bloom
Citizens United for
Research in Epilepsy

Scotty Bowman
Abbott Laboratories

Robin Brumlow
Epilepsy Foundation of Michigan

Kelly Buckland
Idaho State Independent
Living Council

Cheryl H. Bullard
South Carolina Department of
Health and Environmental Control

James J. Cereghino
Oregon Health Sciences University

Stephanie Dubinsky
Kelsey Research Foundation

Rick Fair
Ortho-McNeil Pharmaceuticals

Elizabeth Flores
Austin, TX

Stacy Folkins
Epilepsy Foundation of Washington

F. Mitchell Garrett
Epilepsy Foundation of
South Alabama

Donald J. Goodwin
South Carolina Department of
Health and Environmental Control

Frances H. Graham
MINCEP Epilepsy Care
National Association of
Epilepsy Centers

Margaret J. Gunter
Lovelace Clinic Foundation

Kathy Hampton
GlaxoSmithKline

Linda Harris
Niceville, FL

W. Allen Hauser
Columbia University

Dale Hesdorffer
G.H. Serigevsky Center

E. Wayne Holden
Opinion Research Corporation
Macro International

Lewis Holmes
Massachusetts General Hospital

Margaret Jacobs
National Institute of
Neurological Disorders and Strokes

Andres M. Kanner
Rush-Presbyterian St. Luke's
Medical Center

Amy Kosloski
Epilepsy Foundation of Colorado

Chris Koutsogeorgas
Epilepsy Foundation of
South Carolina

Allan Krumholtz
University of Maryland
Medical Center

Linda D. Lanier
The Sarcoidosis Awareness Network

Kimford J. Meador
Georgetown University Hospital

Chris Merritt
Epilepsy Foundation

Georgia D. Montouris
Boston University School of Medicine

Kathleen Morris
Wyckoff, NJ

Christer E. Osterling
American Epilepsy Society

Karen Parko
Northern Navajo Medical Center

Alexis Perlmutter
Golden, CO

Susan Pietsch-Escueta
Epilepsy Foundation of Los Angeles,
Orange, San Bernardino, and
Ventura Counties

R. Eugene Ramsay
University of Miami
School of Medicine

Tina Robinson
Stockbridge, GA

Michael Rogawski
National Institute of
Neurological Disorders and Stroke

Cara Schmitt
Epilepsy Foundation

Paul Scott
National Institute of
Neurological Disorders and Stroke

Anbesaw W. Selassie
Medical University of South Carolina

Shlomo Shinnar
Montefore Medical Center

Susan Spencer
Yale University School of Medicine

Michael R. Sperling
Thomas Jefferson University Hospital

David Thurman
Centers for Disease Control
and Prevention

Edwin Trevathan
Washington University
School of Medicine

Linda K. Warner
Epilepsy Foundation
Board of Directors

Kim West
Epilepsy Foundation of the
Chesapeake Region

Christopher S. Williams
Wilford Hall United States Air Force
Medical Center

Marshalynn Yeargin-Allsopp
Centers for Disease Control
and Prevention

Mark S. Yerby
North Pacific Epilepsy Research

Workgroup C
Self-Management

Workgroup C Co-Chairs

Colleen DiIorio
Emory University School of Medicine

Mary Macleish
Epilepsy Foundation of Arizona

Workgroup C
Background Presenters

Colleen DiIorio
Emory University School of Medicine

Mary Macleish
Epilepsy Foundation of Arizona

Kate Rollason
The ARC of the United States

Patricia Osborne Shafer
Beth Israel Deaconess Medical Center

Workgroup C Members

Lynda A. Anderson
Centers for Disease Control
and Prevention

Gregory L. Barkley
Henry Ford Health System of Detroit

Cynthia Boddie-Willis
Massachusetts Division of
Community Health Promotion

Kelly Buckland
Idaho State Independent
Living Council

Merle Buckland
Idaho State Independent
Living Council

Janice M. Buelow
Indiana University School of Nursing

Jean Collins
Epilepsy Foundation of
Southern New York

Thomas Creer
Ohio University

Sally Crudder
Centers for Disease Control
and Prevention

Patricia K. Crumrine
Children's Hospital of Pittsburgh

Jim Davies
Epilepsy Foundation of
Greater Chicago

Patricia Dean
Comprehensive Epilepsy Program of
the Neuroscience Center at the
Miami Children's Hospital

Colleen DiIorio
Emory University School of Medicine

Ann Donnelly
Miramar, FL

Angela Dutton
Epilepsy Foundation of Western Ohio

Alexandra Finucane
Epilepsy Foundation

Tracy Glauser
Children's Hospital Medical Center
Cincinnati, OH

Kathy Gores
Epilepsy Foundation of
Greater North Texas

Sheryl Haut
Albert Einstein College of Medicine
Yeshiva University

Eric Joice
Epilepsy Foundation of New Jersey

Richard Kahn
American Diabetes Association

Edna Kane-Williams
Epilepsy Foundation

Amy Kosloski
Epilepsy Foundation of Colorado

Eugenie Z. Lindahl
Bellisse, LLC

Mary Macleish
Epilepsy Foundation of Arizona

Roy C. Martin
University of Alabama at
Birmingham Epilepsy Center

James W. McAuley
Ohio State University
College of Pharmacy

Cynthia McCormick
National Institutes of
Neurological Disorders and Stroke

Merle G. McPherson
Services for Children with
Special Health Needs Division
Maternal & Child Health Bureau,
Health Resources & Services
Administration

Jane Meyer
Epilepsy Foundation of
South Central Wisconsin

Robert J. Mittan
North Carolina Epilepsy Center

Nancy Nielsen
American Medical Association

Kevin Oliver
Epilepsy Foundation of Los Angeles,
Orange, San Bernardino, and
Ventura Counties

Bob Pinkerton
Epilepsy Foundation of Colorado

Michael Pramuka
Western Psychiatric Institute and
Clinic of the University of Pittsburgh
Medical Center

Kate Rollason
The ARC of the United States

Tracy Salazar
Epilepsy Foundation of
San Diego County

Nancy Santilli
Elan Pharmaceuticals

Patricia Osborne Shafer
Beth Israel Deaconess Medical Center

Donna Stahlhut
Epilepsy Foundation of
Southeast Texas

Linda Sullivan
Dallas, TX

John Thompson
Epilepsy Foundation of Minnesota

Christine Toes
Finding a Cure for Epilepsy and
Seizures (f.a.c.e.s.)

Kristin Tomek
Epilepsy Foundation of
Western Wisconsin

Workgroup D
Quality of Life –
Impact and Outcomes

Workgroup D Co-Chairs

Frank Gilliam
Washington University
School of Medicine

Peggy J. Walls
Epilepsy Foundation of Kansas and
Western Missouri

Workgroup D
Background Presenters

Joan K. Austin
Indiana University School of Nursing

John J. Barry
Stanford University Medical Center

Lauren Beck
Parents Against Childhood Epilepsy

David Ficker
University of Cincinnati
Medical Center

Selena Fuller
Epilepsy Foundation of
Eastern Pennsylvania

Frank Gilliam
Washington University
School of Medicine

Bruce P. Hermann
University of Wisconsin
Medical Center

Darla Templeton
Epilepsy Foundation of the
St. Louis Region

Workgroup D Members

Raul Ahumada
Epilepsy Foundation of
Central and South Texas

Margarita Anaya
Epilepsy Foundation of Los Angeles,
Orange, San Bernardino, and
Ventura Counties

Joan K. Austin
Indiana University School of Nursing

Debra Babcock
National Institutes of Mental Health

John J. Barry
Stanford University Medical Center

George Thomas Beall
Ogilvy Public Relations Worldwide

Lauren Beck
Parents Against Childhood Epilepsy

Peter Bloom
Citizens United for
Research in Epilepsy

Bill Clayton
Ann Arbor, MI

Tony Coelho
Epilepsy Foundation
Board of Directors

Sandra Cushner-Weinstein
Children's National Medical Center

Manny De La Hoz
Epilepsy Foundation of
Eastern Pennsylvania

David W. Dunn
Indiana University

Guiseppe Erba
University of Rochester Medical Center

Brian Feldman
The Edison Group

Robert T. Fraser
University of Washington
Regional Epilepsy Center

Peggy Friel
Epilepsy Center Swedish
Medical Center

Selena Fuller
Epilepsy Foundation of
Eastern Pennsylvania

Pat Gibson
Bowman School of Medicine
Wake Forest University Baptist
Medical Center

Frank Gilliam
Washington University
School of Medicine

James Santiago Grisolia
Scripps Mercy Hospital

Bruce P. Hermann
University of Wisconsin
Medical Center

Deborah Hirtz
National Institute of
Neurological Disorders and Stroke

Rosemarie Kobau
Centers for Disease Control
and Prevention

Mary Frances Laverdure
Center for Medicare &
Medicaid Services

June Lipsky
Epilepsy Foundation of Long Island

Sharon McMinn
Arkansas Epilepsy Education Association

Nancy Michel
Penn State Neurology Adult
Medical Services

Jennifer Osborne
Epilepsy Foundation of Kentuckiana

Denise L. Pease
Epilepsy Foundation
Board of Directors

Jennifer Raviv
PhRMA

David Ridings
Epilepsy Foundation of Rochester-
Syracuse-Binghamton

Nancy Ridings
Epilepsy Foundation of Rochester-
Syracuse-Binghamton

Sonya Saldana
Xcel Pharmaceuticals

Ann Scherer
Epilepsy Foundation

Sheri Smith
Ramsey County, Minnesota
Board of Public Health

Colleen Stack
Epilepsy Foundation of
Kansas and Western Missouri

Amanda Stansfield
Seattle, WA

Darla Templeton
Epilepsy Foundation of the
St. Louis Region

William H. Theodore
National Institute of
Neurological Disorders and Stroke

William R. Turk
Nemours Children's Clinic
Wolfson Children's Hospital

Ann Van Cott
Veterans Affairs Pittsburgh
Healthcare System

Peter Van Haverbeke
Epilepsy Foundation

Joseph Velenzano, Jr.
Exceptional Parent Magazine

Linda Wallace
Epilepsy Foundation of Connecticut

Peggy J. Walls
Epilepsy Foundation of
Kansas and Western Missouri

Georgina Watkins
Corning, NY

Arnulfo Zamora
Denver, CO

Jeffrey Zirulnick
Epilepsy Foundation of South Florida

APPENDIX D:
Conference Agendas and Speakers

WEDNESDAY, JULY 30, 2003

Plenary Session

Epilepsy and Public Health
- Robert J. Gumnit, MD, MINCEP Epilepsy Care
- Patricia Osborne Shafer RN, MN, Beth Israel Hospital

Epilepsy and Public Health Discussion Panel
- Suzanne M. Smith, MD, Centers for Disease Control and Prevention
- Cynthia Boddie-Willis, MD, Massachusetts Division of Community Public Health Promotion
- Cynthia McCormick, MD, National Institute of Neurological Disorders and Stroke
- Deborah Jones-Saumty, PhD, American Indian Associates
- Merle McPherson, MD, Health Resources and Services Administration
- Panel Moderator: Solomon L. Moshe, MD, Albert Einstein College of Medicine

Epilepsy: The CDC Perspective and Response
- Virginia S. Bales Harris, MPH, Centers for Disease Control and Prevention

Workgroup Meetings
- Workgroup A: Early Recognition, Diagnosis and Treatment
- Workgroup B: Epidemiology and Surveillance
- Workgroup C: Self-Management
- Workgroup D: Quality of Life – Impact and Outcomes

Workgroup A:
Early Recognition, Diagnosis and Treatment

Recognition/Diagnosis
- Phillip Gattone, Epilepsy Foundation of Greater Chicago
- Gregory L. Holmes, MD, Neurology, Dartmouth Hitchcock Medical Center
- Susan Axelrod, Citizens United for Research in Epilepsy

Reactor Panel
- Santi K.M. Bhaghat, MD
- John Booss, MD, Veterans Administration Connecticut Healthcare Systems
- Jeffrey Levi, PhD, George Washington University Medical Center
- Suzanne M. Smith, MD, Health Care and Aging Studies Branch, Division of Adult and Community Health, Centers for Disease Control and Prevention

Access to Care/Treatment
- Jacqueline A. French, MD, The Neurological Institute, University of Pennsylvania
- Susan Eik Filstead, Susan Eik Filstead Stroke and Epilepsy Foundation, Inc.

Reactor Panel (see above)

Worktables with Facilitators
- Recognition/Diagnosis: Implementation – Christine L. O'Dell RN, MSN, Montefiore Medical Center
- Recognition/Diagnosis: Evaluation – Brien J. Smith, MD, Henry Ford Hospital
- Access to Care/Treatment: Implementation – Arlene S. Gorelick, Epilepsy Foundation of Michigan
- Access to Care/Treatment: Evaluation – James C. Cloyd, PharmD, University of Minnesota College of Pharmacy

Workgroup B: Epidemiology and Surveillance

Children
- Edwin Trevathan, MD, MPH, Washington University School of Medicine

Elderly
- R. Eugene Ramsay, MD, University of Miami School of Medicine

Minority Groups
- Dale C. Hesdorffer, PhD, G.H. Sergievsky Center, Columbia University

Socioeconomic Status
- Charles E. Begley, University of Texas School of Public Health

Special Topics (SUDEP, Mortality, etc)
- Michael R. Sperling, MD, Thomas Jefferson University Hospital

Reactor Panel
- Linda D. Lanier, The Sarcoidosis Awareness Network
- Anbesaw W. Selassie, PhD, Medical University of South Carolina
- David Thurman, MD, Centers for Disease Control and Prevention
- Marshalynn Yeargin-Allsopp, MD, Medical Epidemiologist, Centers for Disease Control and Prevention

Worktables
- Incidence and Prevalence
- Outcomes (i.e survival and mortality)
- Patterns of Care

Workgroup C: Self-Management

Update Since Living Well I
- Patricia Osborne Shafer, RN, MN, Beth Israel Deaconess Medical Center

Self Determination Models
- Kate Rollason, The ARC of the United States

Self-Management Models
- Colleen DiIorio, Emory University School of Medicine

Interventions/Lessons Learned
- Mary Macleish, Epilepsy Foundation of Arizona

Reactor Panel
- Lynda A. Anderson, PhD, Centers for Disease Control and Prevention
- Merle Buckland, Idaho State Independent Living Council
- Sally Crudder, Hematologic Diseases Branch, Centers for Disease Control and Prevention
- Richard Kahn, PhD, American Diabetes Association

Worktables with Facilitators
- Kelly Buckland, Idaho State Independent Living Council
- Janice M. Buelow, RN, PhD, Indiana University School of Nursing
- Jim Davies, Epilepsy Foundation of Greater Chicago
- Eugenie Z. Landahl, Bellisse, LLC
- Roy C. Martin, PhD, University of Alabama at Birmingham Epilepsy Center
- Michael Pramuka, PhD, Department of Psychiatry, University of Pittsburgh Medical Center, Western Psychiatric Institute and Clinic

**Workgroup D:
Quality of Life – Impact and Outcomes**

Epilepsy – A Personal Challenge
- Selena Fuller, Epilepsy Foundation of Eastern Pennsylvania

Overview: Health-Related Consequences of Epilepsy
- David Ficker, MD, University of Cincinnati Medical Center

Health-Related Psychological Consequences and Their Impact on the Individual
- John J. Barry, MD, Stanford University Medical Center

Introduction – The Parenting Challenge
- Lauren Beck, Parents Against Childhood Epilepsy

Psychological Consequences and Their Impact on Health
- Bruce P. Hermann, PhD, University of Wisconsin Medical Center

Epilepsy and the Need for Health Resources
- Darla Templeton, Epilepsy Foundation of the St. Louis Region

Stigma: Observed Health Effects of Stigma on Individuals and Families
- Joan K. Austin, RN, DNS, FAAN, Indiana University School of Nursing

Stigma: Public Health Response and Re-Evaluation
- Frank Gilliam, MD, MPH, Washington University School of Medicine

Reactor Panel
- Sandra Cushner-Weinstein, RPT, LCSW-C, Children's National Medical Center
- Rosemarie Kobau, MPH, Centers for Disease Control and Prevention
- Denise L. Pease, Epilepsy Foundation Board of Directors
- William H. Theodore, MD, National Institutes of Neurological Disorders and Stroke

Worktable Groups – Initial Discussion
- Mental Health – John J. Barry, MD
- Personal Health – David Ficker, MD
- Learning and Cognition – Bruce P. Hermann, PhD
- Institutions and Resources – Frank Gilliam, MD, PhD
- Stigma – Joan K. Austin, DNS, RN, FAAN

THURSDAY, JULY 31, 2003

Plenary Session

Summary Reports by Co-Chairs of Workgroups

Remarks
- Tony Coelho, Epilepsy Foundation Board of Directors

Closing
- Eric Hargis, Epilepsy Foundation

APPENDIX E:
Practice Parameters and Resources for Epilepsy Care

Agency for Healthcare Research and Quality (AHRQ), *Management of Newly Diagnosed Patients with Epilepsy.* Evidence Report/Technology Assessment: Number 39. February 2001. www.ncbi.nlm.nih.gov/books/bv.fcgi?rid= hstat1.chapter.55359.

Agency for Healthcare Research and Quality (AHRQ), *Management of Treatment-Resistant Epilepsy.* Evidence Report/Technology Assessment: Number 77, May 2003. http://www.ncbi.nlm.nih.gov/books/bv.fcgi?rid=hstat1a.cha pter.11665.

American Academy of Pediatrics: Committee on Quality Improvement, Subcommittee on Febrile Seizures. Practice Parameter: long-term treatment of the child with simple febrile seizures. *Pediatrics.* 1999;103:1307-1309.

American Academy of Pediatrics: Provisional Committee on Quality Improvement, Subcommittee on Febrile Seizures. Practice parameter: the neurodiagnostic evaluation of the child with a first simple febrile seizure. *Pediatrics.* 1996;97:769-775.

Ashwal S, Russman BS, Blasco PA, et al. Practice parameter: diagnostic assessment of the child with cerebral palsy: report of the Quality Standards Subcommittee of the American Academy of Neurology and the Practice Committee of the Child Neurology Society. 2004; 62:851-863.

Chang BS, Lowenstein DH. Practice parameter: antiepileptic drug prophylaxis in severe traumatic brain injury: report of the Quality Standards Subcommittee of the American Academy of Neurology. *Neurology.* 2003;60:10-16.

Chronic Disease Directors. The role of public health in addressing lower prevalence chronic conditions: the example of epilepsy. McLean, Va: The Association of State and Territorial Chronic Disease Directors; 2003.

Engel J Jr, Wiebe S, French J, et al. Practice parameter: temporal lobe and localized neocortical resections for epilepsy: report of the Quality Standards Subcommittee of the American Academy of Neurology, in association with the American Epilepsy Society and the American Association of Neurological Surgeons. *Neurology.* 2003;60:538-547. Erratum in: *Neurology.* 2003;60:1396.

French JA, Kanner AM, Bautista J, et al. Efficacy and tolerability of the new antiepileptic drugs, I: treatment of new-onset epilepsy: report of the Therapeutics and Technology Assessment and Quality Standards subcommittees of the American Academy of Neurology and the American Epilepsy Society. *Epilepsia.* 2004;45:401-409.

French JA, Kanner AM, Bautista J, et al. Efficacy and tolerability of the new antiepileptic drugs, II: treatment of refractory epilepsy: report of the Therapeutics and Technology Assessment and the Quality Standards subcommittees of the American Academy of Neurology and the American Epilepsy Society. *Epilepsia.* 2004;45:410-423.

Glantz MJ, Cole BF, Forsyth PA, et al. Practice parameter: anticonvulsant prophylaxis in patients with newly diagnosed brain tumors: report of the Quality Standards Subcommittee of the American Academy of Neurology. i2000;54:1886-1893.

Heck C, Helmers SL, DeGiorgio CM. Vagus nerve stimulation therapy, epilepsy, and device parameters: scientific basis and recommendations for use. *Neurology.* 2002;59(suppl 4):S31-S37.

Hirtz D, Ashwal S, Berg A, et al. Practice parameter: evaluating a first nonfebrile seizure in children: report of the Quality Standards Subcommittee of the American Academy of Neurology, the Child Neurology Society, and the American Epilepsy Society. *Neurology.* 2000;55:616-623.

Hirtz D, Berg A, Bettis D, et al. Practice parameter: treatment of the child with a first unprovoked seizure: report of the Quality Standards Subcommittee of the American Academy of Neurology and the Practice Committee of the Child Neurology Society. *Neurology.* 2003;60:166-175.

Mackay MT, Weiss SK, Adams-Webber T, et al. Practice parameter: medical treatment of infantile spasms: report of the American Academy of Neurology and the Child Neurology Society. *Neurology.* 2004;62:1668-1881.

Optional purchasing specifications for services related to epilepsy: a technical assistance document. GWUMC School of Public Health and Health Services. 2002:1-19. http://www.gwhealthpolicy.org/newsps/epilepsy/.

Ozuna J, Sierzant T, Bell T, et al. Clinical Guideline Series: seizure assessment. American Association of Neuroscience Nurses; 1997.

Practice parameter: management issues for women with epilepsy (summary statement): report of the Quality Standards Subcommittee of the American Academy of Neurology. *Epilepsia.* 1998;39:1226-1231.

Practice parameter: management issues for women with epilepsy (summary statement): report of the Quality Standards Subcommittee of the American Academy of Neurology. *Neurology.* 1998;51:944-948.

Quality Standards Subcommittee of the American Academy of Neurology. Practice parameter: a guideline for discontinuing antiepileptic drugs in seizure-free patients – summary statement. *Neurology.* 1996;47:600-602.

Quality Standards Subcommittee of the American Academy of Neurology, in cooperation with the American College of Emergency Physicians, American Association of Neurological Surgeons, and the American Society of Neuroradiology. Practice parameter: neuroimaging in the emergency patient presenting with seizure – summary statement. *Neurology.* 1996;47:288-291.

Shevell M, Ashwal S, Donley D, et al. Practice parameter: evaluation of the child with global developmental delay: report of the Quality Standards Subcommittee of the America Academy of Neurology and the Practice Committee of the Child Neurology Society. 2003; 60:367-80.